# The Child in Fashion
## 1750 to 1920

Kristina Harris
Photographs by Mare Yaroscak

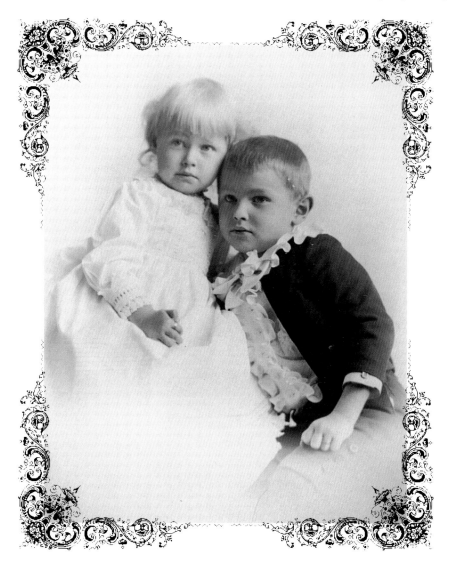

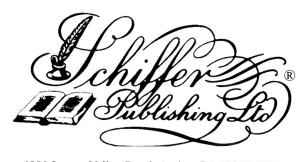

Schiffer Publishing Ltd

4880 Lower Valley Road, Atglen, PA 19310 USA

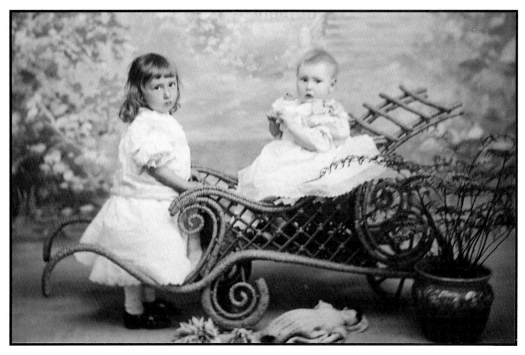

A picturesque scene from the turn of the century. It was difficult to photograph children in the
19th century, since the then modern photographic process required that subjects remain perfectly
still. This accounts for the rather sulky faces of these children, and possibly for the doll that has
been thrown aside to the bottom of the image.

Published by Schiffer Publishing Ltd.
4880 Lower Valley Road
Atglen, PA 19310
Phone: (610) 593-1777; Fax: (610) 593-2002
E-mail: Schifferbk@aol.com

In Europe, Schiffer books are distributed by Bushwood Books
6 Marksbury Avenue Kew Gardens
Surrey TW9 4JF England
Phone: 44(0)181-392-8585; Fax: 44(0) 181-392-9876
E-mail: Bushwd@aol.com

Please visit our web site catalog at www.schifferbooks.com or write for a free catalog. This
book may be purchased from the publisher. Please include $3.95 for shipping. Please try your
bookstore first. We are interested in hearing from authors with book ideas on related subjects.

A Buster Brown style
ensemble, from the pages
of *The Delineator*, 1904.

# Contents

A bodice from the 1860s that
was probably worn by a boy.
*Courtesy of Vintage Silhouettes.*
$120—$275.

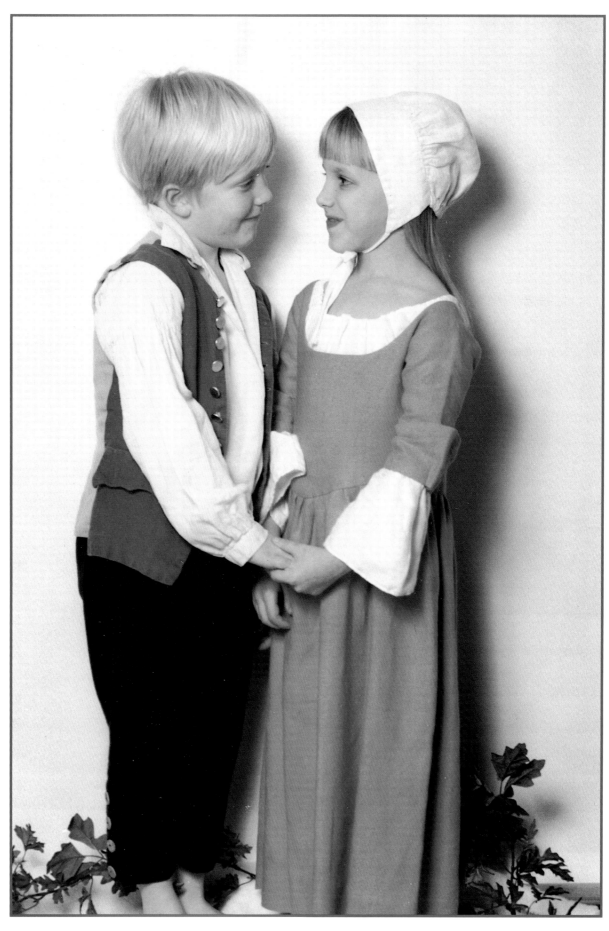

Reproduction 18th century children's attire. Adults wore exactly these same styles.
*Courtesy of Susan Edholm.* Boy's ensemble $189—$240; girl's ensemble $145—$175.

# Acknowledgments

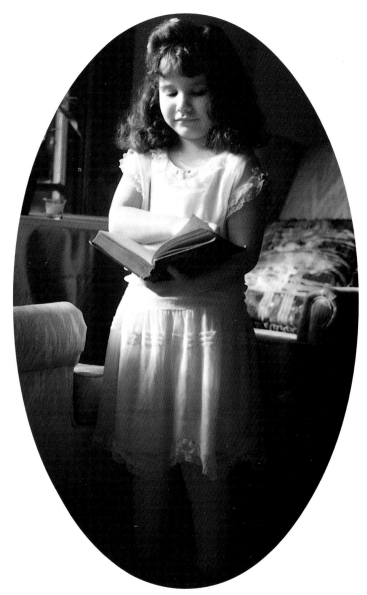

A girl's party dress from the 1920s.

For loaning clothing and accessories from their collection or shops, we thank:

Susan Adholm for her wonderful reproductions of 18th century garb;

Donna Burns, proprietor of *Amazing Lace* in Chatham Massachusetts for loaning from both her private collection and her shop stock;

Pam Coghlan, whose personal collection is shown in part in this book, but who is also the proprietor of a children's and adult's antique/vintage clothing business: *Odds & Ads* in Rutherford, New Jersey;

Janene Fawcett, proprietor of *Vintage Silhouettes* in Crocket, California for sharing generously;

Fay Knicely, proprietor of *Antique Apparel* in Acworth, New Hampshire, for responding generously to last minute requests;

Rosetta Hurley, proprietor of *Persona Vintage Clothing* in Astoria, Oregon, for her ever-enthusiastic participation;

*Mother & Daughter Vintage Clothing* in Waukesha, Wisconsin, for many lovely items;

Laura Hauze Russell, proprietor of *The Cat's Pajamas* in Milville, Pennsylvania;

The Very Little Theatre in Eugene, Oregon, for loaning from their antique and vintage clothing collection;

and to Lucy Sullivan for all her help over the years.

We also give hearty thanks to our young models (and to their parents) for all their patience and enthusiasm. Thank you:

Lily Giannone
Darcie Jones
Christina Lobo
Mackenzie Swan
Natalie Swan
Zachary Swan
Carmen Fraijo
and Jennifer Yaroscak.

A very special thank you also goes to Myra Plant and all of the gracious staff at The Campbell House in Eugene, Oregon, for allowing us to shoot on location. Not only is this bed and breakfast inn a delight to behold, but no one could ask for more friendly people or more courteous service. Thank you!

And finally—but perhaps most importantly—I thank all those readers who asked: "What about a book on children's clothes?"

In the 19th and early 20th century, even children wore gloves. *Courtesy of Mother & Daughter Vintage Clothing.* $10—$30.

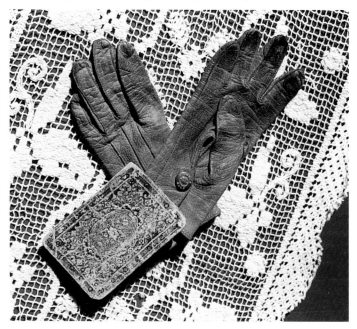

# Author's Note

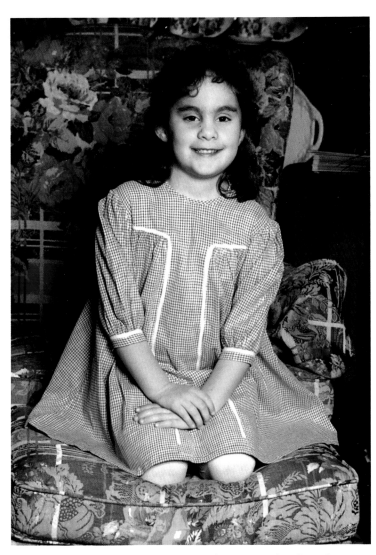

This style of dress was popular in one form or another from the early 1800s through the 20th century. This dress happens to date to the 1920s. *Courtesy of The Very Little Theatre.*

*L*ike many thoughtful people in the field of historical fashions, Mare and I believe in the conservation of clothing as artifacts; we also acknowledge the fact that wearing historical clothing leads to the destruction of these important historical artifacts. Nonetheless, Mare has photographed many of the garments in this book by having them modeled on live persons. If we seem to contradict ourselves, let me explain.

We believe that clothing, like other artifacts, is best appreciated if it is well presented; and there is no better way to present the value, craftsmanship, and beauty of historical clothing than as it was intended to be seen—on a live figure.

For those like us who are concerned with the clothing's health, we assure you that no article was worn by a model if it was in an especially fragile state. Unlike a fashion show, Mare's photo sessions allowed ample (supervised) time for the models to get in and out of the garments with care. No garment was worn for more than a few minutes, and all garments were always carefully protected.

In fact, because these garments were worn only briefly, they were probably in less danger of harm than garments mounted on mannequins and displayed for an exhibition.

Kristina Harris

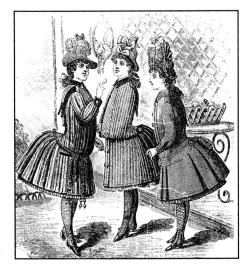

Fashionably dressed girls from the 1870s. Most little girls did not wear such exaggerated bustles.

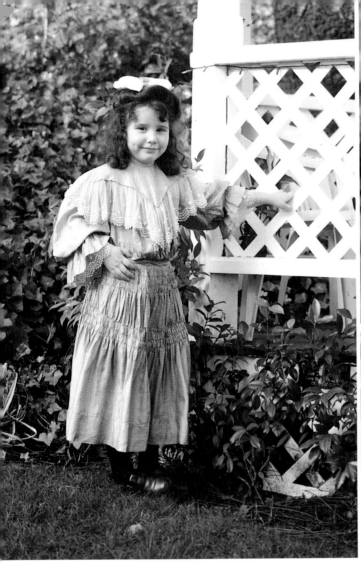

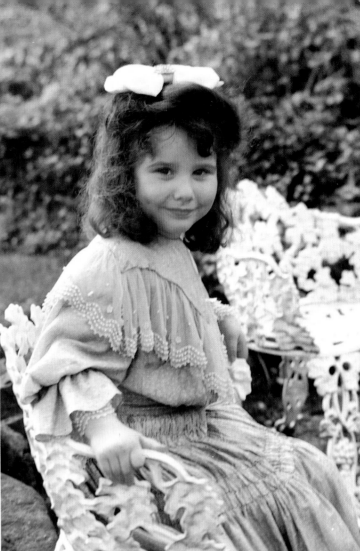

Dresses like this one of silk embellished with lace, ruffles, and smocking, were typical attire for girls in the early 1900s. *Courtesy of Vintage Silhouettes.* $125—$300.

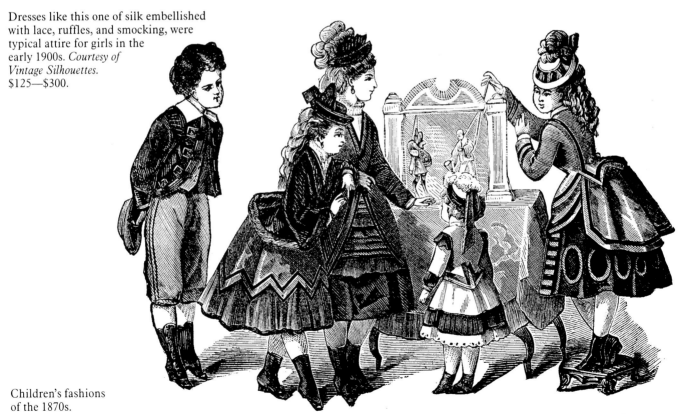

Children's fashions of the 1870s.

# Introduction

The story of children's clothes is the story of childhood itself.

Why did children look like miniature adults until the mid–18th century? Why were little boys clothed in dresses until fairly recent years? Why did babies sometimes wear corset–like garments? The answers to these and many more questions provide a rich history of the childhood experience—explored through the most intimate of historical artifacts: Clothing.

Even more so than adult fashions, childrens' fashions are inextricably tied to outside forces. Whereas adults can presumably choose what they wish to wear, children are dressed by their parents (and consequently, their parents' desires and goals for their children play a large part in how children are dressed). Comfort—perhaps the thing considered most important in childrens' clothing today—was usually the last consideration in children's clothes of the 18th, 19th, and early 20th centuries. More often, politics, elitism, and even influences as seemingly sweet and benign as storybooks and school life have influenced the way children dress. The history of children's clothing is an amazingly detailed tapestry, with threads that lead in many different directions.

Rather than giving a detailed run-down of hem lengths and sleeve styles, I have tried to pick up many of the more intricate tapestry threads and weave them into this book. School systems, coming of age ceremonies, relentless training of little girls to become housewives, and the reasons behind corsets and swaddling...all of these are reasons behind children's fashions that provide more insight to styles than a mere timeline of dress or suit styles. No single book could cover every facet of historical childrens' fashions; but here we hope to help you explore this intriguing world in a new light, whether you are a collector of children's clothes or simply curious about the evolution of childhood.

"A certain, dear, old–time mother used to give her children a dose of nauseous medicine when they quarreled, to sweeten their disposition, she said. A half teaspoonful of compound tincture of gentian, put into a little water, and administered with due solemnity, might have a soothing effect upon the temper even these modern days." *Home & Health, 1907*

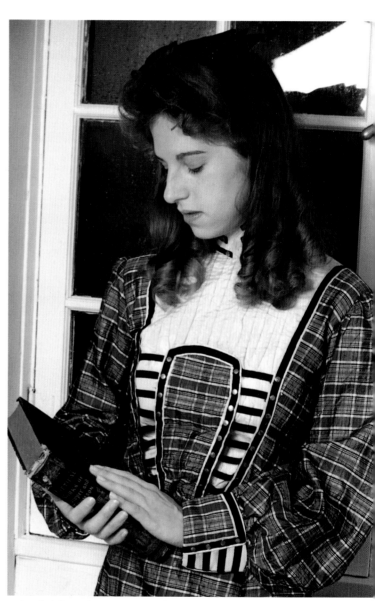

A miss' dress from the turn of the century. *Courtesy of Vintage Silhouettes.*

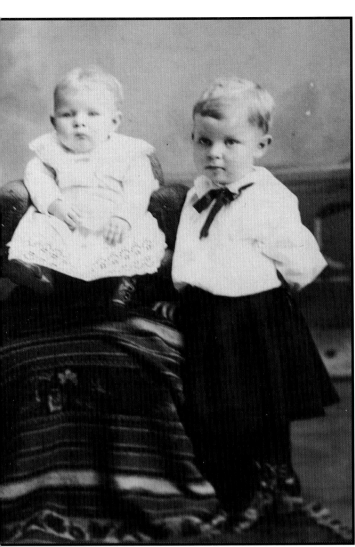

"Little Polly Flinders
Sat among the cinders
Warming her pretty little toes;
Her mother came and caught her,
Whipped her little daughter
For spoiling her nice new clothes."

Typical mid–19th century children's attire.

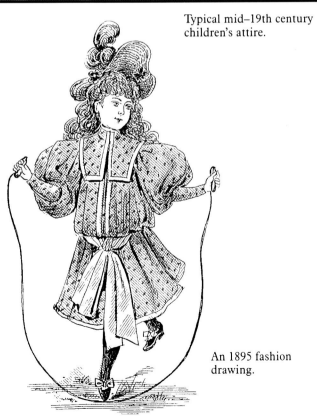

An 1895 fashion drawing.

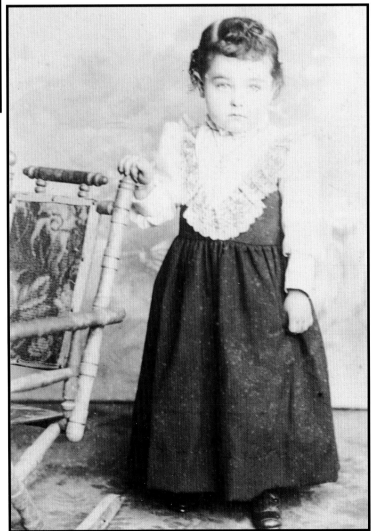

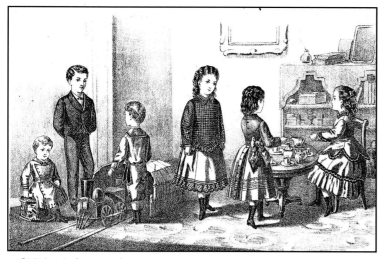

Children's fashions from an 1873 *Metropolitan* fashion plate. $50—$75.

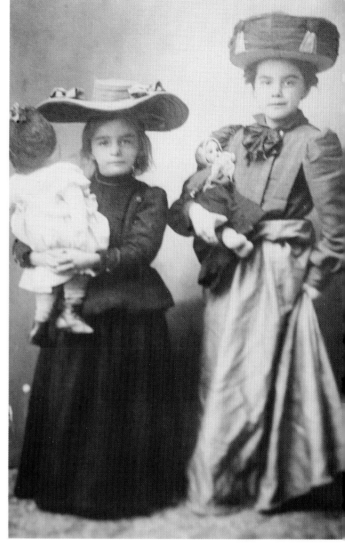

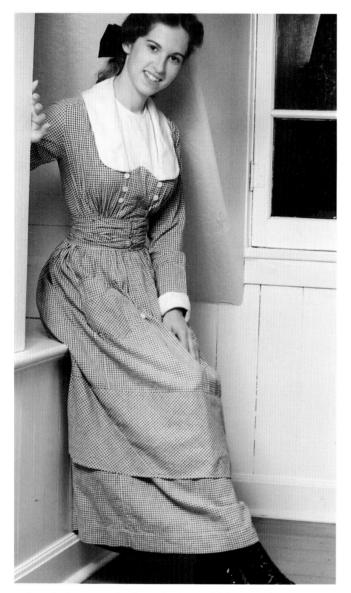

A typical young miss from the 'teens. This style of dress, made of checked cotton with the wide waistband, slim skirt, and white collar and cuffs was practically a uniform for teenage girls during this era. *Courtesy of Vintage Silhouettes.* $100—$250.

A rare candid photograph from the 1890s, showing two little girls playing "dress–up."

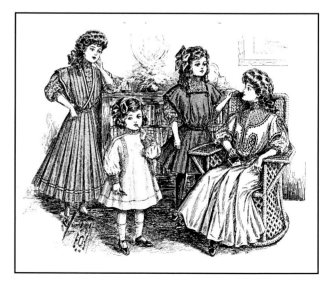

Girls clothing from 1908.

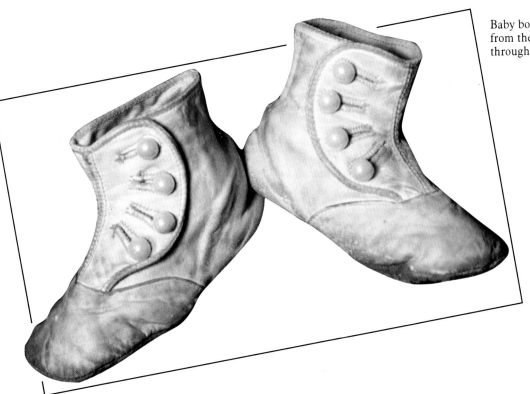

Baby boots like these were worn from the late 19th century through the 1920s. $10—$35.

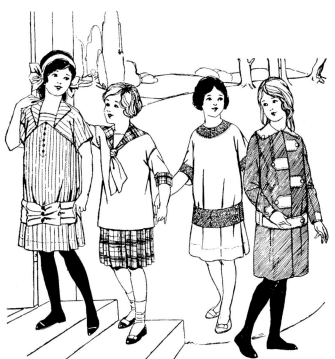

Girls 'teens era dresses, showing definite geometric styling.

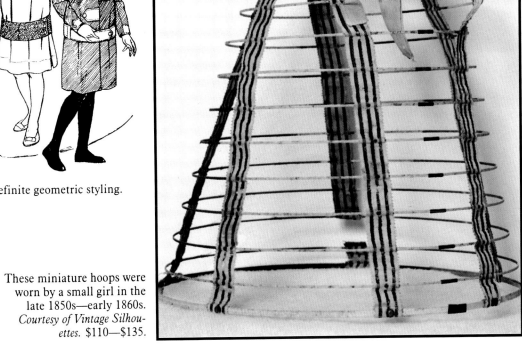

These miniature hoops were worn by a small girl in the late 1850s—early 1860s. *Courtesy of Vintage Silhouettes.* $110—$135.

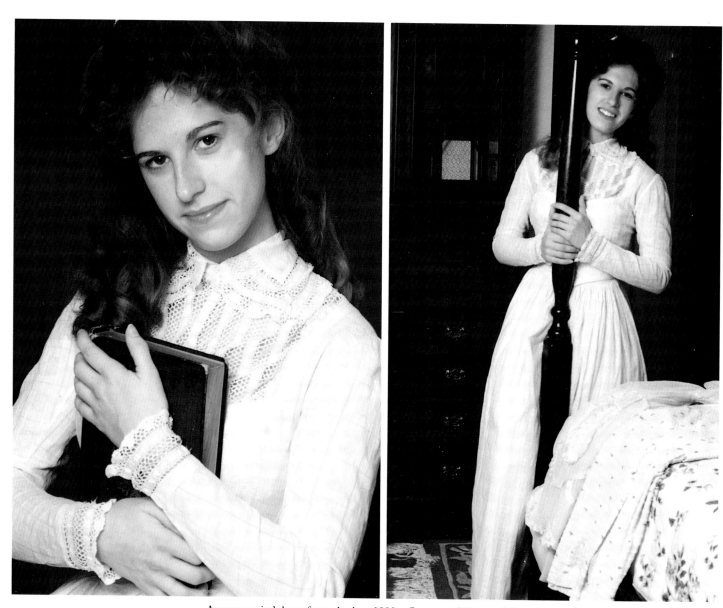

A young miss' dress from the late 1880s. *Courtesy of Vintage Silhouettes.*

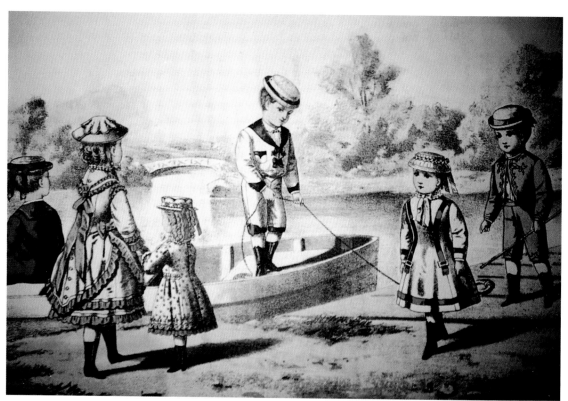

Children's fashions from the early 1870s. $50—$75.

# The Revolution: From Miniature Adults to Children

Children's clothing was invented in the mid-18th century—a mere 250 years ago.

It wasn't, of course, that children didn't wear clothing before this time; on the contrary, they often wore quite a lot of it. But the mid-18th century was the first time children weren't dressed as miniatures of their parents—the first time clothes designed for the special needs of childhood were developed.

For the first time, the idea that children were *not* just mini-adults took flight. Great thinkers and social reformers presented the idea that children were unique from adults in many ways; they were more fragile, they argued, and were more innocent—novel ideas at the time. For the first time *ever* in history, the concept flourished that children ought to have special diets in order to make them grow into stronger, healthier adults, and that—significantly—their clothing should reflect all of these new notions.

A 1778 fashion plate of a middle–class woman and her young daughter. The girl wears a corset and pannier under her woolen dress, a purely ornamental, striped gauze apron, a grown–up style straw hat, and carries a walking stick. $75—$125.

What was this revolution in children's clothes really like for children themselves? The typical attire of fashionable children in the 18th century, before social reforms, was stifling. Reminiscing of her 18th century childhood, Johanna Schopenhauer recalled her typical formal attire:

"An enormous tower of hair, supported by a contraption of wire and horsehair and crowded with masses of feathers, flowers and ribbons, added at least an *ell* to my height; the little white stilts, hardly more than an inch thick, which I wore beneath by ball shoes decorated with gold–embroidered ribbons, sought to redress the balance at the other end of my little person; but although they came nowhere near the height of the headdress, they were nevertheless high enough only to allow me to touch the floor with the tips of my toes. A tightly constructed harness of whalebone–sticks, sufficiently firm and stiff to withstand a bullet, violently pushed back arms and shoulders, pushed the chest forward and constricted the waist about the hips to wasp-like proportions.[1]"

18th century girls also often wore "leading strings," an accessory popular since the 16th century. These were just what they sound like: strips of fabric with one end sewn to the dress at the shoulders and the other end allowed to fall down the back freely. (Those strings that were not sewn directly onto clothes could be pinned on.) Apparently, these strings were often

This is not to say, however, that change was even as quick as the slow and bloody process of over-turning a government—something mid- and late-18th century society was all too familiar with. Children still worked if they came from working-class backgrounds; not infrequently, girls became wives at twelve or slightly older; many boys went to work for their fathers at seven or eight years old; numerous boys left home at thirteen; and children were still held up to the adult standard when it came to social behavior.

"A boy is an appetite with a skin pulled over it." *Anonymous*

practical—especially for younger children—and were used as a leash; but even as children grew into their teens they often continued to wear leading strings, and such strings soon became a symbol of a girl's station in life. To say a girl was "in leading strings" was to say that she was still a child and under her mother's care—not yet fit for marriage.

Up until the mid-18th century, boys, too, could wear leading strings, but only as toddlers. That these were a boon to busy mothers seems clear. "Pray desire Cousen Peg to by me a pair of leading strings for Jak," one woman wrote in a letter dated 1715, when her son was nearly four years old. "There is stuf made on purpose that is very strong for he is so heavy. I dare not venture him with a comon ribin."[2] Using a "string" or leash as long as five feet was a fairly common practice, for both young boys and girls. There is also some evidence that mothers may have actually tied their children up to trees and fences with these strings, while their own hands were busy with the enormous task of keeping house in the 18th century.

More than most people realize today, children of middle and upper class families had wardrobes of variety. By the mid- to late 18th century, a school boy could own a dozen shirts, eight grown-up styled cravats, six snug waistcoats, six pairs of tightly fitted breeches, hats, gloves, stockings, handkerchiefs, and heeled shoes. He might also bring to school a sewing kit that included basic supplies for repairing his expensive clothing. Similarly, a typical girl in boarding school owned a dozen or so dresses (varying in splendor) for various occasions, a decorative quilted petticoat, a decorative hat, a hooped petticoat, a decorative apron or two, a cloak, a corset, heeled shoes, stockings, gloves, handkerchiefs, and a sewing kit.

Though minus the obligatory girl's corset and hoopskirt, boys' clothing was restrictive, featuring snugly–fitted breeches, heeled shoes, and a jacket tight at the waist and around the arms. But previous to the 1750s or so, people saw no reason children's clothing should offer any more freedom than adult clothing. In fact, unlike Johanna Schopenhauer, many people writing of the clothing they wore as a child in the 18th and 19th centuries noted that while their clothes were frequently impractical and uncomfortable, they provoked a feeling of being well–dressed—giving pride, confidence, and a sense of being gown–up.

Noting this phenomenon, one woman wrote in a letter dated 1785 that "Miss P. came over. She is grown quite a young woman...her hair dressed without powder and a linnen gown with a small hoop..."[3] Girls from fashionable families could wear hoops and powdered wigs as young as three, and little boys were complete miniatures of their fathers—but whatever discomfort this created, it was considered worthwhile by many.

Go-carts (which were remarkably like today's baby walkers) served much the same purpose as leading strings, but by the late 18th century, both contraptions were being condemned. "Go-carts and leading strings not only retard the increase of a child's activity, and produce an awkwardness of gait very hard to be corrected afterwards, but often affect the chest, lungs, and bowels, in such a manner as to pave the way for habitual indigestion...or consumptive complaints," wrote Dr. William Buchan in his *Advice To Mothers*.[4] Writer and reformer Jean Rousseau also had his say about the matter; children, he pronounced, "shall have...no leading strings."[5]

By the 1760s, leading strings were worn only by fashionable girls as decorative and symbolic accessories—and even then, only on more formal clothing. After all, as one woman wrote in 1759, "they only dirty and look trolloping" otherwise.[6] Still, it would seem that mothers who had no servants to tend to the endless duties of housekeeping allowed the use of practical leading strings to continue; as late as 1870, one etiquette book condemned the practice as "apt to cause the ugliest deformities, the sinking of the neck between the shoulders."[7]

It was in the 1740s that an Englishman named John Locke wrote the first book attempting to steer parents toward children's clothing specially designed for childhood. Little came of this first effort, but in 1762, when a little volume titled *Emile* was published, the first mass changes could be seen. Written by Jean Jacques Rousseau, *Emile* found instant success in the author's home country of Switzerland and was translated to English in 1763. The rest of the world was less enthusiastic about Rousseau's book, and though Rousseau himself acknowledged the more respected Locke as his inspiration, *Emile* was considered controversial enough to be banned in some countries. Jean Rousseau also became the subject of hearty debate. Not only were his ideas on raising children thought radical and subversive, but they seemed counterfeit coming from a man who had abandoned his five illegitimate children to a Parisian foundling hospital. Though Rousseau later claimed he abandoned his children for their own good (it was impossible to write and to support them at the same time, he said), these actions made it difficult for even Rousseau's most staunch supporters to defend him and his ideas.

Nonetheless, Rousseau's ideas *were* gradually adopted and, considering his low status in the 18th century world, without any help from him. The world was changing, after all. The aristocracy that had for centuries ruled the Western world was loosing its firm grip. Americans were battling the English for freedom from the Monarchy; in France, after decades of growing hatred toward the French aristocracy, the middle class rose up and executed King Louis, Marie Antoinette, and their royal children. The wealthy class in much of Europe was astounded by these bloody revolutions—and fearing their own status (if not their own lives), the aristocracy began to fall away to the background and allow a rising middle class to gain unheard of power and freedom.

*Endnotes:*

[1] *Pictorial Encyclopedia of Fashion*, p.581
[2] *Children's Costume In England*, p.130
[3] Ibid, p.110
[4] *Advice To Mothers*, 1809
[5] *Emile*, 1762
[6] *Children's Costume In England*, p.128
[7] *The Bazaar–Book of the Household*, p.78

Wee Willie Winkie runs through the town,
Upstairs and downstairs in his nightgown.
Rapping at the windows, crying at the lock,
Are the wee ones in their beds, for it's now eight o'clock?"

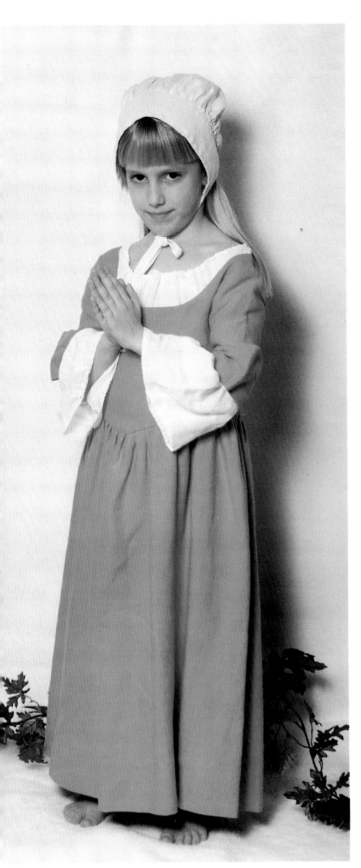

A girl's reproduction dress typical of the 1740s–1760s, featuring a pointed waistline, full skirt, and wing–cuff sleeves. The gown closes with back lacing and is worn with a proper chemise and bonnet. *Courtesy of Susan Edholm.* Ensemble $145—$175.

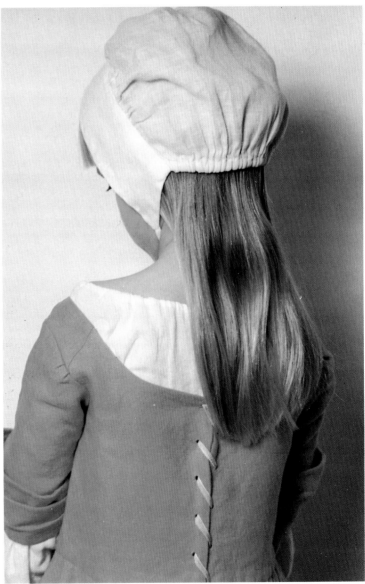

# Making Children Upright

*A*fter centuries of the aristocracy's rigid, counterfeit attire and often unscrupulous lifestyle, a new naturalness was desired to fit in with this new way of life. The garb of country and working class children—more practical out of necessity (just as adult working class people's clothes tended to be compared to the fashionably wealthy people's)—were now adopted for children of all classes.

This "Age of Sensibility" began to emerge just as the sculptures of Herculaneum and Pompeii were re-discovered. Finding the clothing on these Grecian statues fresh and sensible, people of the late 18th century tried to duplicate it. Thinking (incorrectly, as it turned out) that these beautiful Grecian works of art revealed that the ancients dressed only in white, this became the new fashionable color; sheer, flowing, white muslin dresses—first for children and later for grown women—became the height of fashion. The new white children's dresses also lent themselves well to the newly emerging idea that children were gifts from Heaven—*and* the sheer fabrics these dresses were fashioned of also lent themselves well to an old idea: hardening.

"Hardening," or the idea that children needed to be hardened both physically and mentally in order to survive in the world, first became a widespread idea in 1693 when John Locke wrote *Some Thoughts Concerning Education*. Children were often left to run about without shoes, hats, cloaks, and other protective clothing because this was thought to help them build up a resistance to harsh weather and disease.

The new white dresses had other advantages, too. Unlike the old style of rigid, splendid, fashionable clothing, these little dresses were perfectly washable. In fact, it may even be that the washable white, fairly plain baby dresses that had been popular previous to any revolution in children's clothing may have been the more important inspiration for the new muslin dress. For centuries, babies wore cotton and silk gowns with short puffed sleeves, rounded necklines, and high waists—an exact description of the new style of dress, except that now a sash was added to hide the seam between the bodice and skirt. This idea is supported by the fact that at first only toddlers wore the muslin dress while, later, older children (and finally women) gradually adopted the style.

The muslin dress—despite its supposed simplicity—was still, however, a status symbol. Only children from wealthy families could afford the true gauzy, unlined muslin dress. Muslin was primarily imported from India at the time, and it was not inexpensive. Still, less wealthy children benefited from the style, too. Though their dresses were usually fashioned out of printed cottons or wools, they still found relatively free movement in the simple cut of the dress. Nonetheless, the white dress was more prevalent among the less fashionable classes than might first be suspected. "One pretty daughter [of a shoemaker], a light delicate fair–haired girl of fourteen...See her on a Sunday in her simplicity and her white frock, and she might pass for an earl's daughter," wrote Mary Russell Mitford in a story for *Ladies' Magazine*.[1] The difference between the shoemaker's daughter's dress and a wealthy child's dress, would have been obvious to their contemporaries, however; a wealthy child wore gauze–like, sheer muslin, while the shoemaker's daughter could only afford a more opaque cotton.

I personally remember as a child of seven or eight, looking through the family photo album and, upon finding a sepia–toned photo of a toddler in a white, lace–trimmed dress, being told it was my grandfather. "Grandpa!" I was shocked and even giggled at the thought of my dad's dad donning a dress. But this is purely a modern perspective, and it's important to remember that the muslin dress worn in the late 18th and early 19th century was not delegated to girls alone—boys also wore dresses during this period. "The limbs of a growing child should be free to move easily in his clothing," Rousseau wrote in *Emile*, offering up the common reasoning for keeping both boys and girls in skirts. "Nothing should cramp their growth or movement...The best plan is to keep children in frocks as long as possible and then to provide them with loose clothing, without trying to define the shape which is only another way of deforming it."[2] It was a theory that would not die easily.

Trousers—as opposed to fitted breeches—were virtually unknown as the 19th century opened. The first inklings of the acceptance of trousers was in the late 18th century, when girls donned drawers under their flimsy white dresses. From about 1790 to 1810, these undergarments varied, as no doubt many styles were tested before a standard was set. Sometimes they were open-crotched, with a narrow waistband being the only thing holding the two legs together. Other times, they were closed in front (and sometimes even in the back) and had side buttons—which must have been the most modest for childhood play. More peculiar were drawers with legs that were not attached at all: they were two separate tubes that tied at the knee—or sometimes at the waist. This style was short-lived, since the tubes tended to slip or completely fall

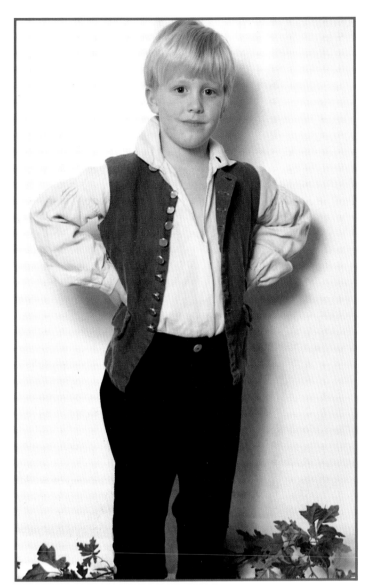

This reproduction ensemble is typical of boy's clothing from 1750–1770s. The shirt is loose–fitting; the breeches have a buttoned fall front, knee cuffs, vents on the sides of the legs, and are laced to fit the waist in back. The vest (or weskit) also laces up the center back. *Courtesy of Susan Edholm.* Ensemble $189—$240.

began testing the waters with full–length trousers—though they were by no means mainstream. It seems that like the entire revolution of children's clothing, trousers have their beginnings in peasant clothing. One theory is that Marie Antoinette, when she was desperately trying to gain the favor of France by dressing herself more like a peasant, had a portrait painted of her children. Her eldest son—who was supposed to become king—dressed in trousers for this 1785 painting. Still, like Marie Antoinette's own wearing of the chemise dress (a predecessor of the muslin dress seen at the turn of the century) this must have been sneered upon. But Marie Antoinette was not the only one touting the country theme. Rousseau did also, and even Sir Walter Scotts' family was painted in 1815 dressed in peasant–like clothing. Yet while boys may have been accepted in trousers by the early 1800s, when the Duke of Wellington arrived at the fashionable

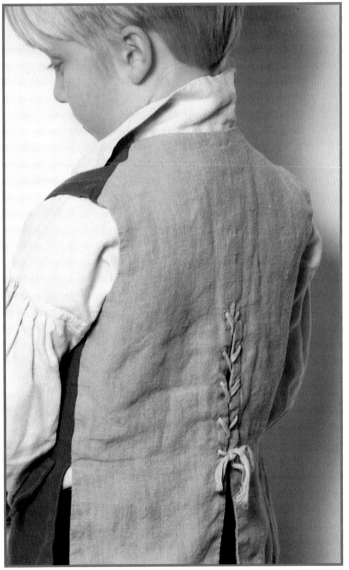

off. Interestingly, while some modern writers have claimed that this latter style was used only by children from poorer families, some existing examples are of the expensive variety—made of fine fabrics and trimmed with lush laces. It seems much more likely, then, that this style was adopted because it made the drawers seem less like masculine trousers.

By the early 1800s, drawers were an accepted part of children's wear. "It is now so much the fashion to dress children, both boys and girls, in pantaloons instead of petticoats," *The Lady's Economical Assistant* advised in 1808.[3] Skirts were too slim to make movement possible in more than a single petticoat—but the sheer muslin dress required a little more modesty than a lone petticoat could provide. (It wasn't until the late 1850s that drawers for adult women became widely popular.)

Like the muslin dress, and like drawers, children wore trousers before adults ever did. In the 1780s, boys tentatively

"Almanak's" club in 1814 wearing trousers rather than breeches, he was refused entry—despite his prestige.

"I've no *baby* now!" Katherine Bragdon wrote in her 1869 diary, when her son was three years old. "Put pants and a little blouse on my little Darling Boy. He looks as sweet and cunning as need be and is as proud and happy a little lad as ever wore pants and is so careful not to soil them by getting on the floor..."[4] Just when a boy should be breeched—that is, switched from dresses into trousers—was a matter hotly debated throughout the late 18th and 19th century. It was not unusual for "experts" to claim that breeching shouldn't be done before the age of eight. But most often, the advice given was that age had little to do with it—size matter more. Though the exact timing was generally left up to mothers, the general consensus was that breeching should come before it was too late. "Her disposition, with her natural feminine tastes and tenderness, is always inclining her to deck her child with the gewgaws of finery and coddle him with the delicate appliances of luxury," one 19th century book opined. "The timely check from the manly boy may therefore prevent her from persisting in an effeminating process which would be sure, if continued, to deprive him of his best characteristics."[5]

Yet at whatever age breeching took place, it was considered a joyous event—and a sign of growing manhood. "Being four and a half years old," wrote William Hutton, speaking of his breeching in the 1720s, "and dressed in my best suit, a cocked hat and walking stick my sister took me by the hand to Gilbert Bridge's for the evening milk, which in the future was to be my errand. One of his buxom daughters in a gay mood snatched off my hat...I gave her a blow with my stick; she returned the hat."[6] Family celebrations coinciding with breechings were not uncommon, and breeching parties are often mentioned in dairies. "You cannot believe the great concerne that was in the whole family here last Wednesday, it being the day that the Taylor was to helpe to dress little Frank in his breeches in order to the making an everyday suit by it," wrote Anne, Lady North in a letter dated 1678.[7]

At least one poem was written about the important breeching event:

> Joy to Philip, he this day
> Has his long 'coats cast away,
> And (the childish season gone)
> Put the manly breeches on.
> Sashes, frocks, to those who need'em—
> Philip's limbs have got their freedom.[8]

Occasionally, girls were mentioned as having been breeched—but this referred only to their underwear, in days when drawers were sometimes still thought crude for girls. In a letter dated 1824, Sara Hutchison wrote: "I am sorry to hear that little dear Good–Good has been breeched—for some of the faculty opine that it is much better that females should not—and Mary H. gave up the practice of putting her Girls into Trowsers from her own experience that it was injurious."[9]

While the idea that 18th century children were forced into corsets from a very early age may make modern parents wince, this was one area where the new relaxed standards in children's clothing did not change. From the 18th century though much of the 19th century, children—boys and babies,

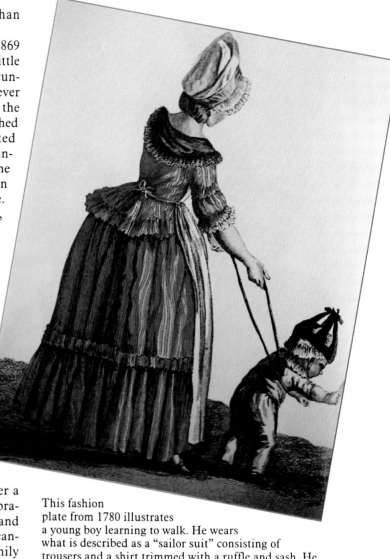

This fashion plate from 1780 illustrates a young boy learning to walk. He wears what is described as a "sailor suit" consisting of trousers and a shirt trimmed with a ruffle and sash. He also wears a type of pudding cap (described as a *bourrelet*), and is firmly held by his governess by the aid of leading strings. $75—$125.

in addition to girls—wore some form of the corset. A child's first corset could be given to him or her when just a baby; these were never boned, but were constructed of firm cotton, and were quilted or corded for strength. Boys were allowed to doff these snugly–fitted bodices once they were breeched, and sometimes as soon as they could walk. Though it seems most likely that these early, unboned corsets were intended to keep children warm, some 18th century reports indicate that when a child did not stand or sit properly erect, knitting needles were inserted into their otherwise unboned corsets to force them into correct posture.

Once girls reached the age of eleven or so, they were usually gradually introduced to corsets with bones. No doubt, another part of the reason girls were made to wear corsets at an early age was so that their first adult corset wouldn't seem like pure torture. Nonetheless, the transition was far from easy—especially when a girl had been allowed total freedom of figure in her early years. This seems to have occurred more often in the United States than anywhere else, and many

American mothers wrote of feeling pity for their girls, wishing that they could continue to let them be free—at least until they hit their teens.

"The first reformation in my appearance was effected by a stay–maker," wrote Elizabeth Hamm of her first real corset in 1793. "I was stood on the window seat whilst a man measured me for the machine, which in consideration of my youth, was to be only what was called half–boned, that is instead of having the bones places as close as they could lie, an interval, the breadth of one was left vacant between each. Notwithstanding, the first day of wearing them was very nearly purgatory, and I question if I was sufficiently aware of the advantage of a fine shape to reconcile me to the punishment."[10]

As the 19th century opened and progressed, the use of corsets on very young children diminished—but many were still forced to wear one on formal occasions. While this new leniency may have made early childhood easier, it made the progression into womanhood much more difficult for girls. Nonetheless, mothers were brainwashed into believing that to not corset their daughter was a great sin. Even as late as the early 20th century, fashion magazines, how–to books, and corset ads touted: "Your child must be kept healthy or she cannot be beautiful."[11] And corsets, by keeping the child warm, her posture correct, and her freedoms in check, accordingly kept her "healthy and beautiful."

"Those mothers who are desirous of giving their daughters slender waists should be careful in the application of the corset," *The Metropolitan* magazine instructed in 1871. "It should fit the figure exactly, but without compression, as the use of a well–fitting corset, though not compressing the waist, will hinder its growth. For children, corsets should be chosen which are low in front, so as not to impede the full expansion of the chest; they should also be high in the back, in order to keep the body upright. After the girl reaches the age of fourteen, the full corset should be worn, when, if the figure does not possess the requisite slenderness of waist, a very slight constriction of the corset will bring it about."[12] This was something of a modern and enlightened view for the era, and only a decade earlier, one mother confessed that her daughter "wore [the stays] the first night after much protestation, but on the second I found she had taken them off after I had retired to rest. I then took the precaution of fastening the lace in a knot at the top of the lace–holes, and for a night or two this had the desired effect; but she was not long before she cut the staylace. I have punished her somewhat severely for her disobedience, but she declared she will brave any punishment rather than submit to the discipline of the corset. She is now fourteen…[and] does not complain that the right–lacing makes her feel ill."[14]

The general consensus was that fourteen was a good age to put girls into full–fledged corsets—which hardly seems coincidental. "The discipline" of the corset was, like the layers upon layers of clothing women and girls wore, a way to help ensure virtue, as well as inactivity. But because many girls of the middle and lower classes never made it into corsets until that age, the corset issue became a subject of hot debate. "I must beg that you will allow me to declare that when stays are not worn till fourteen years of age, very tight lacing causes absolute torture for the first few months," one woman wrote to *The Englishwoman's Domestic Magazine*. She went on the tell the horror–tale of one girl who'd been in boarding school,

*Don'ts For Parents*
1. Don't train your baby to cry for everything in sight, or he will soon learn the value of tears.
2. Don't neglect early training in orderly habits.
3. Don't allow demonstrations of temper. Screaming, kicking, and striking need never be struggled with if 'nipped in the bud.'
4. Don't allow 'whining' or 'teasing.'
5. Don't fail to express sympathy when the child is in trouble. Sympathy is soothing.
6. Don't tolerate talebearing. It breeds selfishness.
7. Don't criticize and punish first, and investigate later. Injustice inflicts a deep wound.
8. Don't offer bribes. Teach obedience from principle.
9. Don't push the little ones from you for fear of their soiling a pretty gown. Sometimes you may long for their caresses.
10. Don't fail to fulfill promises. This will instill confidence.
11. Don't give opportunity for the children to question your justice.
12. Don't fail to be kind and considerate. Kindness is a mighty conqueror.
13. Don't neglect forming the acquaintance of your children's playmates and companions.
14. Don't try to frighten your children into obedience by telling them ghostly tales, or shutting them up in a dark place.
15. Don't fail to require good manners at the table. Habits early formed will stay by children through life.
16. Don't use language that you would blush to hear your children repeat.
17. Don't manifest partiality toward any one of your children. They are keen observers.
18. Don't look for polite answers from your little ones if you fail in this respect. They are excellent imitators.
19. Don't treat your girls and boys in such a careless way that they will bestow their confidence elsewhere. When you lose that, you lose your stronghold.
20. Don't put everything up out of the reach of the baby finger. An understanding that some things are not to be touched will be a good lesson in self–control.
21. Don't turn a child off with an evasive answer when he is seeking special information. He will get it elsewhere.
22. Don't deceive yourself by thinking that your children will grow up to be gentleman and ladies unless you treat them as such.
23. Don't frown and scold the children continually and expect them to be sweet–tempered.
24. Don't feel above making an apology if you have wronged your child. This is one way of establishing confidence.
25. Don't permit your children to stay with their playmates overnight. Be fearful of their learning lessons of impurity.
26. Don't fail to instill honor and truthfulness into their young hearts, by example as well as by precept. To do this under all circumstances requires courage, but it pays." *Home & Health, 1907*

and been tortured by corsets there. In reply, another reader wrote: "[She] is...an exception, for it is seldom that girls are allowed to attain the age of fourteen or fifteen before commencing stays. The great secret is to begin their use as early as possible, and no such severe compression will be requisite. It seems absurd to allow the waist to grow large and clumsy, and then to reduce it again to more elegant proportions by means which must at first be more or less productive of inconvenience. There is no article of civilized dress which when first begun to be worn does not feel uncomfortable for a time to those who have never worn it before. The barefooted Highland lassie carries her shoes to the town, then puts them on upon her arrival, and discards them again directly she leaves the centre of civilization. A hat or a coat would be at first insupportable to the men of many nations, and we all know how soon the African belles threw aside the crinoline [hoop skirt] she had been induced to purchase."[14]

Nonetheless, particularly in the United States, many girls ran about freely, uncorseted, until they reached puberty and both their character and their bodies were considered necessary to reign in. Parents who could afford to do so often gave this unpleasant task to a boarding school, and by the mid–19th century, such schools had a reputation for ruthlessness. One girl who was trained for a corset in this manner complained that corsets "were real instruments of torture; they prevented me from breathing and they dug deep holes into my softer parts on every side."[15]

But girls were not the only children physically hampered. "How has my heart ached many and many a time when I have seen poor babies rolled and swathed, ten or a dozen times round; then blanket upon blanket, mantle upon that; its little neck pinned down to one posture; its head more than it frequently needs, triple–crowned like a young pope, with covering upon covering; its legs and arms as if to prevent that kindly stretching which we rather ought to promote...the former bundled up, the latter pinned down; and how the poor thing lies on the nurses lap, a miserable little pinioned captive," one 18th century novel described the plight of babies.[16] The practice of "swaddling" babies, utilized since the 14th century, was still being regularly practiced in the late 18th century. While today the thought of binding up a baby "as firmly as an Egyptian mummy in folds of linen"[17] seems cruel to most people, there were "good" reasons for the practice.

Though the actual method of swaddling and how the fabric was bound across the body varied over the years, the essential idea behind the practice remained consistent. In 1671 Jane Sharp's *The Midwives' Book* explained the theory aptly: "Infants are tender twigs and as you use them, so they will grow straight or crooked."[18] Swaddling was meant to aid the growth of babies by keeping them straight and healthy. In addition, swaddling was a means of keeping infants out of trouble; there is some evidence that mothers hung their babies on wall pegs while they did their daily housekeeping—a practice little different from women sometimes seen on the evening news today, who hang their children up on walls covered with Velcro. Too, the average household was a much more dangerous place one– or two–hundred years ago. "Baby–proofing" is a modern concept, and in the pre–20th century world, open fires and new–fangled machinery were great dangers to children. Many mothers worked outside the home as well as inside it, and could not stop to pick up the baby every ten

minutes; her only alternative to swaddling then, was to give the child some alcohol to subdue it.

Actual swaddling was more than just a single, firm wrap, however. A shirt, opening in the back, was also worn, in addition to a "bellyband" that was literally wrapped around the belly area. A "napkin" or diaper was also worn, as well as a cap or handkerchief for covering the head. Then, bands of fabric were wrapped around the body of the infant, giving it the look of an ancient Egyptian mummy. By the 18th century, these bands were usually replaced by a single snug cloth, making the baby a neat package. Sometimes another band was added under the head covering and was pinned to the clothing at the shoulder in order to keep the head straight and make movement extremely difficult. Still, after three weeks or so, the baby's arms were generally allowed out from under its swaddling, and in another four months, the baby was freed entirely from it binds.

Yet even parents who might have loathed the thought of actual swaddling did practice the use of rollers—even well into the 1920s. "She took off [the baby's] roller—such many, many times she turned the baby to pull of the long roller!" one Victorian writer exclaimed.[19] Made of a single, straight piece of cloth, some rollers measured as much as ten feet in length, and a roller of eight feet was not uncommon.

Though in 1785 a doctor writing for *Lady's Magazine* claimed that "the barbarous custom of swathing children like living mummies, is now almost universally laid aside," and while John Locke opposed swaddling for political reasons ("The infant is bound up in swaddling clothes, the corpse is nailed down in his coffin," he wrote, comparing swaddling to, in his words, "slavery")[20], as late as the first few years of the early 1900s, some American infants were still being subjected to it—despite the new and more comfortable standards being set for children's clothing. It has been suggested by childhood specialists that there were definite reasons for this prolonged use of swaddling—as well as the early use of corsets, leading strings, and walkers: It made children "upright." From very early on, this word has had dual meaning. Literally it means to stand on two feet, but significantly, it also means having a good sense of morality. By using devices that kept children straight and upright, parents were ensuring that children did not crawl on the floor like mere animals. As one Dr. Francois Muriceau warned Victorian parents, if crawling was allowed, children would always "crawl on all fours like little animals."[21]

But while an infant's swaddling may have had some negative connotations, a babies' christening gown was nothing less than beautiful—figuratively and literally. Long, white, and often quite elaborate, the christening gown represented a ceremony unlike any other. Though it's primarily Catholics that believe in infant christenings (most other Christians believing that a child must be aware of what the ceremony represents before baptism can have any meaning), there is no pagan celebration or ceremony that replaces a christening. Up until the 20th century, a baby's christening was its first appearance in society, and was as much a way to announce the child's birth (and its name) as it was to dub it a Christian. In fact, the christening was such a part of the baby's introduction to society that specific Sunday services were often set aside for christenings, so that all the neighborhood could witness the event.

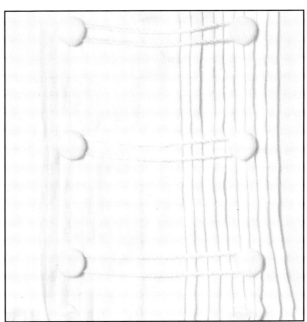

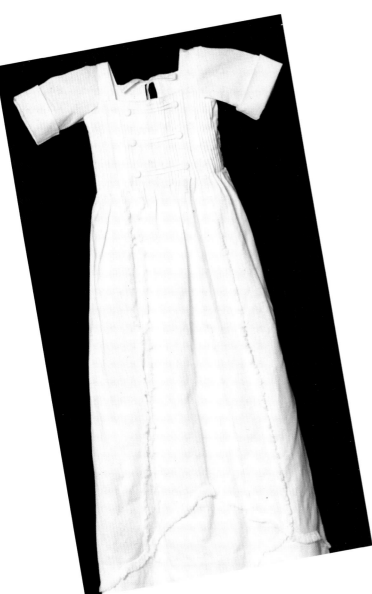

Reproduction baby attire of the 1770s–1790s. "Slip" gowns like these were standard wear for babies, and often featured Hussar trim—two rows of buttons joined with a lacing cord. The trim derives its name from the uniforms of the Hungarian Light Calvary, and was an especially popular trim for boy's clothing of the period. This gown also features self–fringe on the skirt, and ever–popular tucks on the bodice. The gown closes in back with fabric ties. *Courtesy of Susan Edholm.* $290—$300.

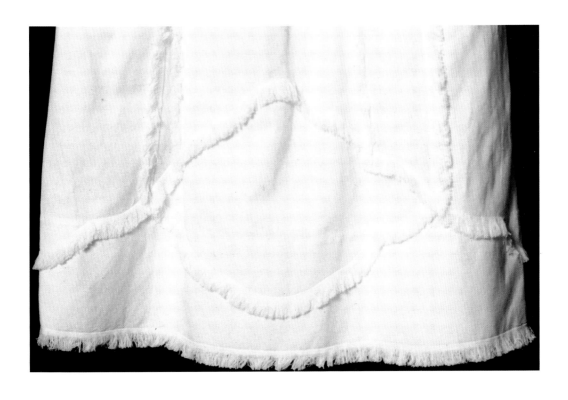

The first mentioning of christenings was in the 3rd century—but the ceremony was by no means commonplace at that time. Up through the 18th century, it was usually midwives—not clergymen—who christened babies. Mortality rates were high, and if the parents believed the child must be christened before it could go to Heaven, it's understandable why a church christening was impractical. Later christenings were still performed promptly after the birth, but were now held in church, becoming a ceremony mothers were physically unable to attend. Tradition had it that babies could wait no longer than three days after their birth to be christened—and within those same three days, the law insisted that the child's father must go to town hall along with two witnesses (usually neighbors) to declare the birth and have it recorded. An official doctor would then verify the birth by visiting the family home—and, amusingly enough, check to make sure the parent's had correctly noted the sex of the child. It actually was not until the Victorian era that mothers insisted on taking part in the christening ceremony and that it was delayed a few weeks for their benefit.

Christenings were also ceremonies full of folk customs. Up until the mid- to lateVictorian era, for example, the baby was often rolled on the alter "to strengthen its muscles and prevent rickets and lameness."[22] Godparents were an essential part of the ritual, also—so much so, in fact, that mothers of illegitimate children often paid for one. The godfather and godmother of the christened babe were supposed to kiss as they passed under the belfry on their way out of the church—but there were other immediate duties as well. "It is a difficult thing to ask people to be godparents," one Victorian writer admitted. "The modern idea that has encrusted the ecclesiastical idea is, that the godfather should present a silver mug, or knife, or fork, or spoon, or something of that kind, and sponsorship becomes a serious tax on one's benevolence."[23] Other attendees were also an essential part of the ceremony, and in France, the children of the town frequently followed in procession after the christening, "raising a terrible racket with hammers and rattles in order to make sure that the child would not grow up deaf and dumb and, in the case of a girl, that she would have a pleasant speaking and singing voice."[24]

The first christenings were performed like baptisms—by dunking or immersing the child in water. After the 8th century, however, sprinkling the child's head with water became an alternative when an infant's health might otherwise be jeopardized. Though the water in baptism represents many wondrous things (the creation, when God put life in the water; the water of the great flood, which gave mankind a new beginning; the parting of the Red Sea that led the Jews out of slavery; the water of the Jordan where Jesus was baptized; the tears of Jesus at his crucifixion; and, ultimately, the behest of Jesus: "Go out and teach all nations, baptizing them in the name of the Father and the Son and of the Holy Spirit"), it was often criticized by doctors as contributing to the high infant mortality rate. In 1831, *The Lady's Book* noted that a Dr. Trevisian, who had researched this topic in Italy, claimed that of 100 babies born from December through February, 68 died in their first month, and 15 more within their first year, leaving a mere 19 to live longer. Further, he claimed, of one hundred children born in the spring, 48 survived their first year; of summer babies, 83 survived their first year; and of autumn children, 58 lived past a year. The cause of their early deaths?

The doctor claimed it was their exposure to water in their christening.

But folklore had other things to say about the water involved in christenings. It was often thought a blessing if the child cried when exposed to the water, since this was supposed to indicate that Satan was being driven away from the child's body. Some folklore even went so far as to say that if a child didn't cry when it was christened, it was too good and Godly to live in human form. "On the 16th our boy was christened," Caroline Clived noted in her diary in 1842. "The ceremony was performed after the morning service and he cried only enough to satisfy his nurse who said she must have pinched him if he had been totally silent because children who don't cry when christened die soon after."[25]

As the sprinkling style of christening became the norm, a "chrism cloth" became a necessary article of attire for the infant. This was essentially a piece of fabric that was placed over the child's head after the sprinkling. Later, an actual cap replaced the chrism cloth, and a chrism gown was used. As early as 1549, prayer books directed clergymen to note this garment during the ceremony: "Take this white venture for a token of innocencie, whiche by Gods grace in this holy sacramente of Baptisme, is given unto thee."[26] The baby then wore this christening gown for three weeks after the ceremony.

Being a "token of innocence," christening gowns, right from the start, were often pure white—but there were exceptions. Because the christening was, in essence, the baby's debut, it was natural for the child's parents to want it to look as darling and well–dressed as possible. Because it was conspicuous, and because it contrasted so well with a new born's fair skin, red was often an early favorite. Satins and velvets trimmed with embroidery, lace, and ribbons were equally popular whether the gown was pure white or scarlet red. Even in the colonial days of America, William Bradford of Plymouth had a gown made for his baby that was crimson silk with embroidered pink and yellow flowers.

With the elaborate christening gown came the outer trappings of mantles, capes, and bonnets. Englishwoman Susan Sibbald wrote that at her sister's christening in 1792, the baby wore "the most beautiful blue and white satin mantle, blue hat and feathers." Later, Charles Dickens wrote of one middle class babe "packed up in a blue mantle trimmed with white fur."[27]

It wasn't until the late 18th century that the long white christening gown came into massive popularity. These were still often satin, decorated with pintucks, lace, ruffles, and about a yard or so long. As the Victorian era appeared, christening gowns varied in length according to the wealth of the parents—some gowns being as long as four or more feet. The idea was that the gown should touch the floor even while the child was being held in the arms of a standing adult. It wasn't until the 1920s that shorter skirts became popular—usually no longer than three feet, and often much shorter. Christening gowns from the 19th century nearly always feature short sleeves; rather low, scooping necklines; and a seam between the bodice and the skirt. It wasn't until the 1870s that the princess line, or dresses without waistlines, appeared.

"Within a few years we have shortened the long clothes worn by youngest infants," one writer proclaimed in 1903. "Twenty–five years ago the handsome dress of an infant, such as the christening–robe, was so long that when the child was held on the arm of its standing nurse or mother, the edge of the robe barely escaped touching the ground."[28] It wasn't until baby carriages were in regular use that christening gowns were shortened considerably. Too, styles in fashion were changing. Where once elaborate clothing was favored, simplicity was coming into vogue. Robings all but disappeared, and many heirloom Victorian gowns were shortened. "One woman ripped off the deep flounce of old Buckinghamshire lace from the second–best christening robe and substituted a frill of coarse machine–made embroidery, saying she was not going to taker her child to church 'trigged out' in that old–fashioned trash. As she had not troubled to unpick the stitches, the lace was torn beyond repair," wrote one woman about a borrowed christening gown.[29]

### Endnotes:

[1] *Our Village*, which was published in book form in 1824
[2] *Emile*, 1762
[3] *Children's Costume In England*, p.197
[4] *Century of Childhood*, p.23
[5] *Bazaar Book of the Household*, p.214
[6] *Children's Costume In England*, p.117
[7] *History of Children's Costume*, p.31
[8] "Going Into Breeches" by Mrs. Leicester; ibid, p.32
[9] *Children's Costume In England*, p.198
[10] ibid., p.128
[11] Warner corset ad, c. 1890s
[12] *The Metropolitan*, July 1871, p.54
[13] *Englishwoman's Domestic Magazine*
[14] ibid.
[15] *Children's Clothing*, p.125
[16] *Children's Costume In England*, p.103
[17] *History of Children's Costume*, p.20
[18] *Children's Clothing*, p.15
[19] *The Diary of a Baby Boy* by E. Berger, p.157
[20] *Children's Costume In England*, p.104
[21] *Century of Childhood*, p.35
[22] *History of Private Life*, p.312
[23] *Welcome Sweet Babe*, p.33
[24] *History of Private Life*, p.312
[25] *Welcome Sweet Babe*, p.44
[26] *Edward VI, Prayer Book*, 1549
[27] Charles Dickens, "Bloomsbury Christening," 1836
[28] *Welcome Sweet Babe*, p.89
[29] ibid., p.91

# Little Visitors

Its eyes are blue and bright,
Its cheeks like rose;
Its simple robes unite
Whitest of calicoes
With lawn, and satin bows.

Thomas Hardy, *The Christening*

*Y*et, it was not only christening gowns that were long and white. "Every article of dress, for a new–born infant, should be white," *Godey's Lady's Book* proclaimed in 1857.[1] This tradition existed partly because of the association of white with purity (though previous to the early 1800s, children were often looked upon as more evil than good); but practicality probably had more to do with the popularity of white than anything else. By keeping the clothes white, rather than colored or printed, mothers ensured that the baby's clothes—which would be soiled daily and require constant washing—would not run or fade as badly as colors and prints did.

Babies did, however, sometimes wear color—particularly to help delineate their sex to onlookers. "If you like the color note on the little one's garments, use pink for the boy and blue for the girl, if you are a follower of convention," one 1914

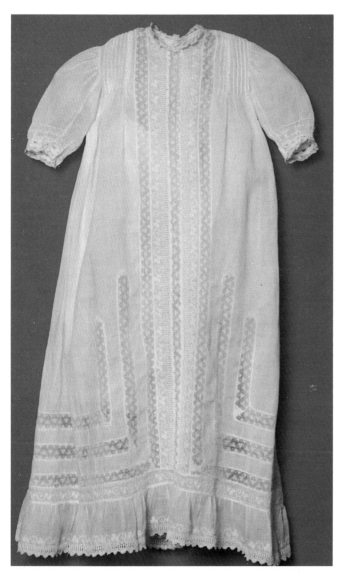

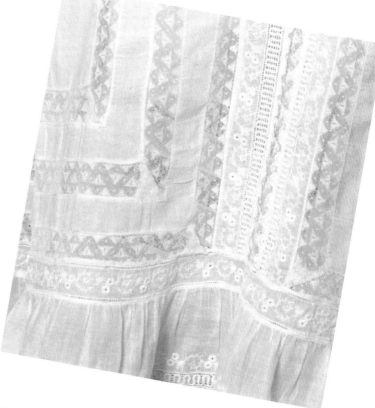

This turn–of–the–century batiste gown was probably worn for a christening. It shows many fine examples of typical christening gown embellishments, including pintucks and lace insertions. The gown closes with two mother–of–pearl buttons in back. *Courtesy of Amazing Lace.* $150—$190.

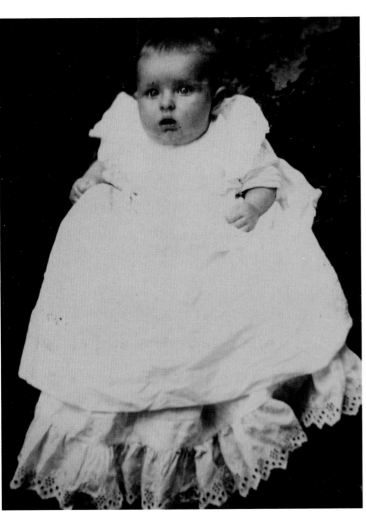

By the late 19th century, babies were frequently photographed in their christening gowns—but not all white dresses were actually christening dresses.

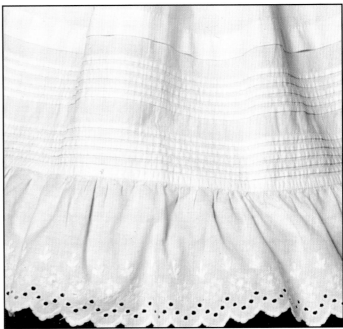

This baby slip originally would have been worn under a christening gown, helping to give a voluminous look. The wide band at top would have come just under the baby's arms. $30—$65.

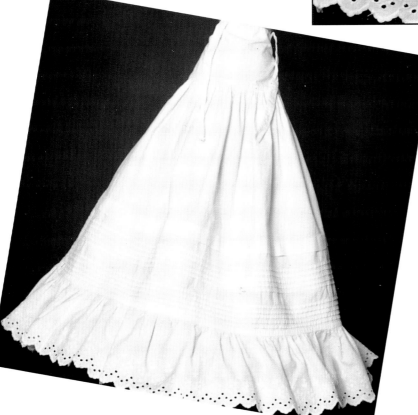

*Life's Lessons*

Along with the basic skills of reading, writing, and arithmetic, a girl's education in the 18th, 19th, and even the early 20th century was not considered complete without lessons in housekeeping: Cooking, cleaning, and sewing. As part of a girl's lessons, the headmistress of her school (or her mother, if she was unable to attend school) required her to complete what was called a "sampler." This was essentially a piece of linen with letters, numbers, verses, and motifs embroidered onto it—but to girls and their families, it symbolized much more.

Originally, the sampler was intended to be a "try-out" for important sewing skills: By cutting out the linen for the sampler, a girl learned to cut fabric accurately and economically. Next, she learned the essential hemming stitch by turning the edges of the cloth and stitching them under. Then she embroidered a decorative border around the piece, using simple, basic stitches that she would use later in life to decorate plain linens like tablecloths, pillowcases, and dishtowels.

The girl then added the alphabet to her sampler; this served a dual purpose. If the girl was quite young, it helped her to learn her alphabet, or to write it out. And since all linens were expensive (made by hand until the third quarter of the 19th century) and were always marked with the owner's initials for identification, stitching the alphabet gave her much needed practice for stitching legible letters. Numbers might then be added to the sampler for the same reasons: In order to learn them, and to learn to stitch them legibly for future use. The rest of the sampler was then filled in with motifs that often included less practical, prettier, "fancy stitches." Still, even these had learning value since they were most often symbols or quotations from the Bible, or poignant reminders of what society expected from a girl's life.

Most samplers were cherished—either by the girl who stitched them (as a reminder of stitches), or by her family members, who would proudly frame and display her sampler in the parlor. The sampler was not only a basic learning tool for girls, displaying the skills that would help make them fine housewives, but samplers also helped direct girls toward their futures. By teaching them never to have idle hands, and to be mindful of what God and society expected of them, samplers were a way of teaching girls to be women.

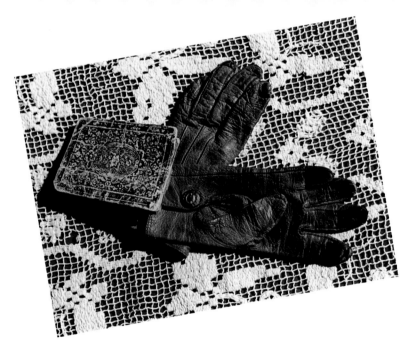

There are a total of 13 miniature sampler charts in this c.1840s–70s hand–size booklet. Measuring a mere two inches wide by three inches long, it was well used by its original owner. The leather gloves are from the turn of the century; each closes with a single "Fownes Make" marked snap. *Courtesy of Mother & Daughter Vintage.* Charts $50—$100; gloves $10—$30.

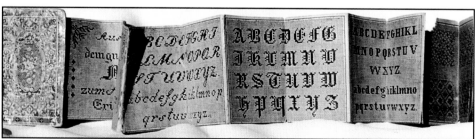

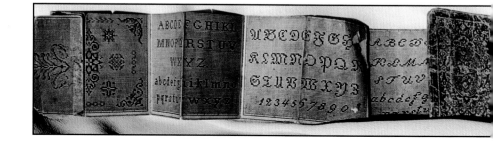

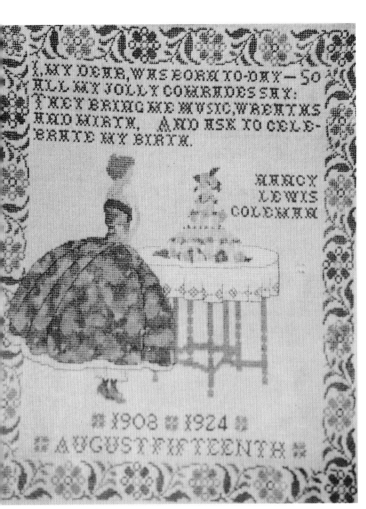

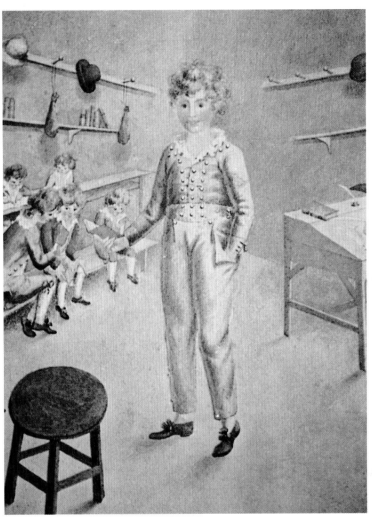

A sampler completed in 1924 by a girl aged 16. $300—$500.

An early 19th century illustration, showing a typical school boy of the period.

*Christened By The Sea*

One of the most wondrous accounts of a christening was given in the 1953 book *O Rugged Land of Gold* by Martha Martin. Martin, who was married to an Alaskan gold prospector, was separated from her husband one winter by a landslide; pregnant, she was left alone to suffice for herself. She broke several bones, but was reunited with her husband in spring, alive and well, and with a new child in tow.

Yet even under these trying circumstances, Martin wrote that her baby, Donnas, was "christened by the side of the sea...Many friends will come to see Donnas baptized, but no relatives will be there, no godparents. Many deer will come, perhaps the ravens will fly over, the jays will be on hand, and a great eagle might look on from a far–off high perch...Donnas was dressed in all her finery and wrapped in the otter robe, only her little face showing deep down in the fur...I carried her proudly to the water's edge, scattered food about, and waited for the deer to come.

'Dearly beloved,' I told my baby and the assembled crowd, 'we are gathered together here in the sight of God and in the face of this company to baptize this child...Almighty and everlasting God, heavenly Father, Lord God of Hosts, we give Thee thanks for all Thy many blessings, the greatest and best of which is the placing of this child in our care...'

Then I knelt down at the edge of the sea and said: 'Donnas Martin, I baptize thee in the name of the Father, and of the Son, and of the Holy Ghost. Amen.'

I dipped the tips of my fingers in the water and signed my child with the sign of the Cross...Then I said the Lord's Prayer, and Baby and I went back to the cabin.[1]

[1] *Sweet Babe*, p.37–38

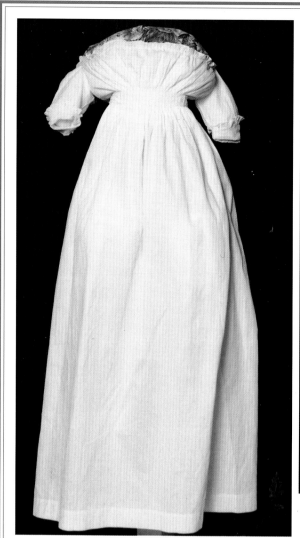

This c.1800–1815 cotton dress features a waistline that lies just under the bust, and is trimmed with a band of whitework. A plain tie wraps around to the back to secure the waist, and two drawstring closures are featured in back. The hand sewing on this dress is so finely executed that it could be mistaken for machine stitching at first look. *Courtesy of Antique Apparel.* $350—$700.

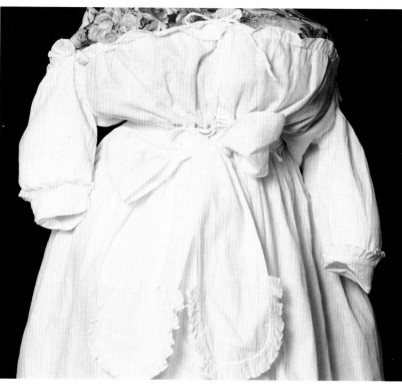

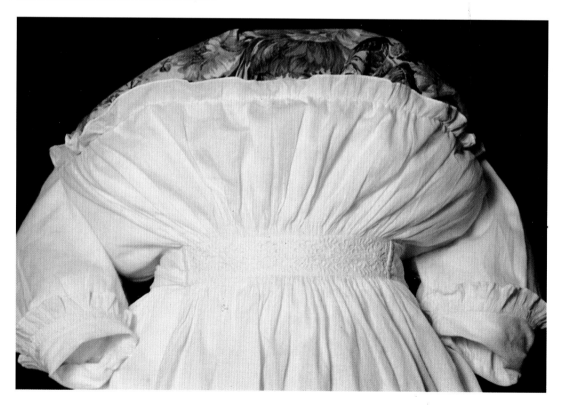

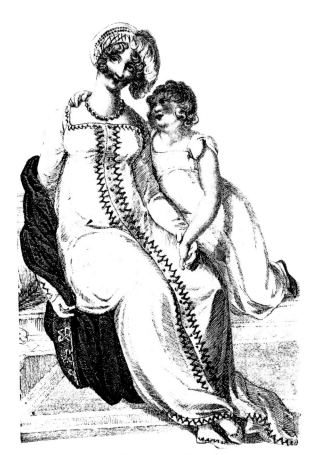

A girl's dress from 1810. It varies little from her mother's, except for the inclusion of a marked (though high) waistline.

---

newspaper article advised. Only a few years later, in 1918, *The Ladies' Home Journal* reported that "There has been a great diversity of opinion on the subject, but," the writer insisted, "the generally accepted rule is pink for the boy and blue for the girl. The reason is that pink being a more decided and stronger color is more suitable for the boy, while blue, which is more delicate and dainty, is prettier for the girl."[2] This reasoning may seem very odd to us today, but the opposite way of thinking did not take firm hold until around World War Two. Pink, being most closely associated with bold, daring red, was considered more masculine, while blue (always an easier color to achieve in dyes) was softer and more subdued. Too, blue is the color associated with the Virgin Mary, and, in the Middle ages, the color of true lovers and faithful servants.

Sometimes babies were dressed entirely in the color associated with their sex. In one journal of 1784, it is noted: "Baby's [attire] was blue and very pretty she did look."[3] But most often, the color was an accent to the costume. More unusual (and probably a short-lived custom) was a special signal on the baby's cap; in 1838 one book noted that "a rosette of satin ribbon is worn on the left side if a boy, and in front, if a girl."[4]

But whether or not the baby's cap was coded for its sex, caps were an essential part of dressing babies up through the 1920s and beyond. Caps were worn day and night—and not infrequently, two at a time. If two were worn, often the first was simple and either plain cotton or wool; the second cap tended to be more ornamental—trimmed with lace, quilted,

embroidered, or otherwise embellished. Very elaborate, decorative caps were designed for christenings—and like the outer cloak, could be brilliantly colored and embroidered. For such elaborate caps, advisors suggested that "for convenience... several pairs of strings should be provided, and instead of sewing them to the bonnet they may be pinned in place with attractive baby pins, so that they may be easily changed."[5]

In the 18th and early 19th centuries, caps were sometimes designed to help re-shape the baby's head if it was thought too pointed. Even well into the 19th century, "experts" often advised new mothers to put "puddings" or padded caps on their children to help cushion their heads in case of a fall. "Pudding" being a synonym for daffy, these caps would seem to have been aptly named, and a common saying was that you wore a pudding cap so that "your brains won't turn into pudding." (Pudding, however, is also an old-fashioned name for a stuffed sausage, so a stuffed and quilted cap would be aptly named after that reference, also.) Babies from wealthy families also sometimes wore actual hats—large plumes and all.

Up until fairly recent years, babies were often called "little visitors;" many parents held their breath until the age of six, when, common wisdom had it, the child was relatively certain of growing into adulthood. Perhaps because of their untimely deaths, some writers—particularly in the 18th and early 19th centuries—wrote of babies as troublesome, sorrow-giving creatures. Many people appear to have believed that children were inherently evil, and it wasn't until the Victorian era that writers began to describe childhood as having "a beautiful credulity, a sort of sanctity, that one cannot contemplate without something of the reverential feelings with which one should approach being of a celestial nature."[6] Perhaps because of those early, rather bitter writings about babies, the modern notion has often been that parents of the 18th and early 19th century did not attach themselves to their children. It is rather incredible that anyone who's been a parent could believe such a notion—and happily, the people of the age prove their own case for parental love. Diaries with mournful entries after a baby's death, poems to deceased babies, and later, memorial photographs and other momentos of lost babies prove that the love from parent to child was just as strong in the 1790s as it is today.

Nonetheless, much more so than today, infant mortality was a bitter reality of life. As late as the 1850s, in New York City, 49% of all deaths were children under the age of five, and in the state of Massachusetts, 24% of the total female population never reached the age of five. The statistics didn't get much better as the century progressed: 26% of women born in 1890 were dead by or before 1910. "The statement is a startling and fearful one, that about one-half of the human race in civilized society die before the age of five years," *The Household Magazine* noted in 1879. "This fact is all the more humiliating, since it is admitted that a similar mortality is not observed in savage life..."[7]

One help to decreasing this high infant mortality rate was the new and rare specialty called pediatrics. This branch of medicine wasn't developed until the late 1870s—but this does not explain the gap between Western society's infant mortality rates and those of other cultures. One contributor to infants' deaths was the way babies were dressed. The average garb of an infant—whether for boy or girl—was a light-weight

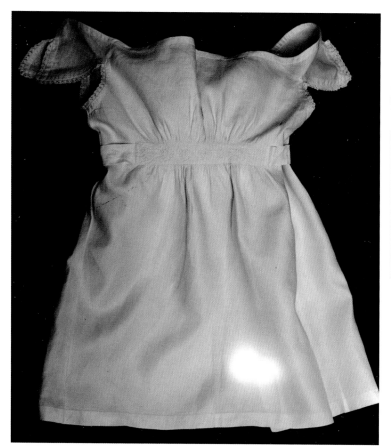

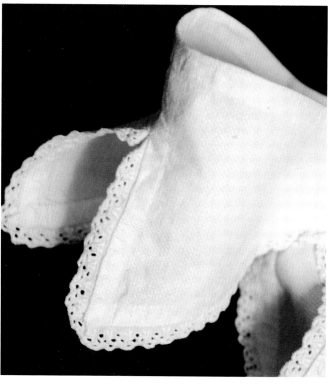

A c.1815–19 baby' dress of cotton. The center whitework band is identical to the older child's dress on page 28. The baby dress also features ties that wrap around the waist and a drawstring at the center top back. This style of epaulet was popular in fashion magazines from about 1818–20. *Courtesy of Antique Apparel.* $250—$400.

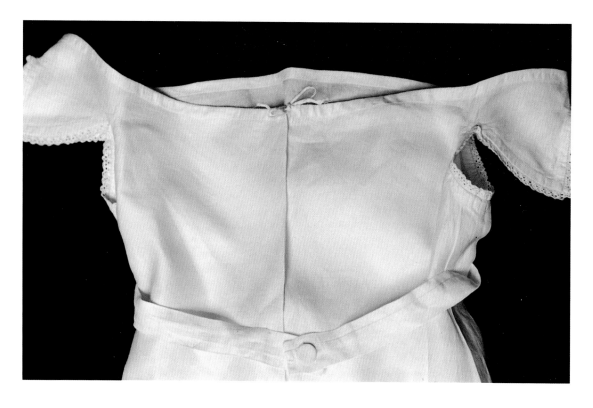

dress with a scooping, rounded neckline, and minuscule sleeves. "The truth is, a new-born infant cannot well be too cool and loose in its dress; it wants less clothing than a grown person in proportion because it is naturally warmer, and would therefore bear the cold winter's night much better than any adult person whatever," doctors advised parents.[8] Even as late as the 1890s, some doctors were still advising parents to keep their babies dressed coolly and to keep them in rooms not exceeding 68 degrees. The idea that babies generated their own warmth was a myth that died hard.

"Very many children are sacrificed, or permanently injured, by the mistaken ideas of mothers on head warmth," *Godey's Lady Book* advised in 1857. Trying to educate mothers, the editors went on to quote "one of the most eminent authorities of the day," one Doctor Bull:

> "Unfortunately, an opinion is prevalent in society that the tender child has naturally a great power of generating heat, and resisting cold; and from the popular error have arisen the most fatal results. This opinion has been much strengthened by the insidious manner in which cold operates on the frame, the injurious effects not being always manifest during, or immediately after, its application; so that, but too frequently, the fatal result is traced to a wrong source, or the infant sinks under the action of an unknown cause. It cannot be too generally known that the power of generating heat, in warm-blooded animals, is at its *minimum* at its birth, and increases successively to adult age; that young animals, therefore, instead of being warmer than adults, are generally a degree or two colder, and, moreover, *part with their heat more readily*. These facts show how great must be the folly of that system of *hardening*.[9]"

Fortunately, even before the majority of parents were educated about this medical fact, some allowances were made for warmer baby clothes. "Where, from circumstances, it may be feared the infant will be delicate, or it is pre-maturely born, and in cold weather, very fine flannel gowns, completely covering even its hands, are very necessary, as warmth will be found one of the most powerful aids in preserving life."[10] In Kate Chopin's 1899 novel *The Awakening*, she tells of one mother who wanted a pattern made for a baby's sleeper; this was "a marvel of construction, fashioned to enclose a baby's body so effectually that only two small eyes might look out from the garment, like an Eskimo's. They were designed for winter wear,

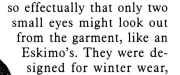

An interesting boy's costume from an 1808 fashion magazine; the style is reminiscent of the skeleton suits that would be at the height of popularity a little later in the century.

when treacherous drafts came down chimneys and insidious currents of deadly cold found their way through keyholes."[11] Indeed, in the days before central heating, it's a wonder more babies did not die more frequently.

For the mother-to-be, sewing the baby's layette—or wardrobe—was an essential task whether she lived in the 18th century or the 1920s. Reading some of the required layettes makes one wonder whether it took nearly all nine months for the sets to be completed, for even during eras when the sewing machine was readily available, nearly every guide advised mothers to hand-sew the tiny articles of clothing. One early layette, from an 1808 book, was listed as:

> Four little shirts
> Four little caps
> Two frocks
> Two little bedgowns
> Two flannel blankets
> Two rollers
> Two pairs of stays and flannel [petti]coats
> Two upper petticoats
> Twenty-four napkins.[12]

In 1838, the layette was more substantial:
> Shirts...12–18
> Flannel bands...2–4
> Flannel caps...2–4
> Night-caps...6–12
> Day-caps...3–6
> Napkins (doz.)...4–6
> Pilchers...4–6
> Pinafores...4–6
> Bedgowns...4–6
> First day-gowns...3–4
> Night-flannels...3–4
> Day-flannels...3–4
> Flannel cloak...1–2
> Flannel shawl...2–3
> Robes...4–6
> Petticoats...4–6
> Socks...4–8
> Hood...1
> Cloak or pelisse...1[13]

In 1913, *McCall's* magazine showed more interest in keeping the infant warm, and listed the minimum requirements as:
> 4 nightdresses
> 4 flannel barrowcoats
> 4 petticoats—flannel
> 2 petticoats—nainsook
> 3 wool or silk and wool shirts—first size
> 3 shirts, second size
> 6 flannel binders, 6 inches by 24, torn from the piece and not hemmed
> 4 dozen diapers
> 1 coat
> 1 bonnet
> 4 flannel jackets
> 2 long flannel or cashmere wrappers
> 1 large shawl
> 1 flannel head shawl.[14]

By the 1920s, Butterick (one of the largest manufacturers of sewing patterns) advised: "All baby clothes should be white, and as fine and dainty as possible. Pale shades of baby pink and blue can be used for ribbons on dresses and caps...Pale pink and blue are also used for baby kimonos, sacks, sweaters and booties, and for afghans, blankets, etc. But the actual dresses, slips, caps and coats, petticoats, etc., are always white...The layette given below is complete and large enough to keep a baby fresh and dainty if one can have constant laundry work done. It is, however, the smallest layette that is safe to start with, and it would be desirable to enlarge it, especially in the matter of diapers, naps and shirts. You must have at least:

> 3 Dresses
> 3 Nightgowns
> 3 Petticoats
> 3 Bibs
> 3 Kimonos
> 3 Sacks
> 3 Knitted Shirts
> 3 Knitted Bands
> 3 Flannel Bands
> 3 Pairs of Booties
> 24 Diapers 18 x 18 ins.
> 6 Quilted Pads 11 x 16 ins.[15]

An unusual 1811 boy's costume from *Repository of the Arts*. The mandarin collar, hat, and parasol all show marked Oriental influence.

But most how–to books and magazines of the period assumed that this somewhat daunting task of creating a babies' layette from scratch was one of great pleasure. "Far more often than we think, the choicest, tenderest thoughts the woman is capable of, and the highest, noblest ambitions of what her baby shall be, and what she shall be to it, are sewed into the little garments with her swiftly flying needle," the author of *What A Young Wife Ought To Know* concluded. [16]

Still, there were many important details for expecting mothers to remember while stitching up their babies' clothing. Most magazines stressed thrift and ingenuity: "Many useful things for baby's use can be contrived by an ingenious mother," *McCall's* advised. "A man's silk handkerchief, for instance, makes an adorable little bonnet. Turn the hem back to give a Dutch effect. This may be embroidered or edged with a crochet edging done in cream silk or simply left plain. Line with cream sateen or silk, and if for a winter baby, interline with sheet wadding."[17]

By the beginning of the 19th century, mothers were primarily asked to consider the infant's comfort and well being. The majority of how–to books of this period condemned the "old–fashioned" style of baby's dress—just as adult–like children's dress had been condemned in the late 18th century. "Formerly the comfort of the baby was little planned for; and more than that, it almost seems, as we consider it to-day, that the clothing of the little one was planned for discomfort...[But] we should consider the baby's comfort, first, last, and all the time. However proud we may be of it we should not allow ourselves to dress it for exhibition. The *baby* is the center of attraction, not what it may be dressed in."[18] Some considerations were more obvious, however. "I open this note to say that we have just discovered the cause of little Fredrick's restlessness," Charles Dickens wrote. "It is not fever, as I apprehended, but a small pin, which nurse accidentally stuck in his leg yesterday evening. We have taken it out, and he appears more composed, though he still sobs a good deal."[19] Unfortunately a cure for ties that wouldn't stay tied and straight pins that poked many a babe would not come until 1878, when the safety pin was first advertised.

"In making your baby–clothes, remember that the infant is constantly growing, and requires, therefore, such clothes as will enable it to move every limb freely. The throat, armholes, and wrists of dresses should be made so that they can readily be let out, besides being amply large for present use," *Godey's* noted in 1857.[20] The length of dresses was also a topic of much debate, some mothers arguing that their child could develop more freely in shorter skirts. While in 1840, a popular guide advised that wealthy children wear 40–inch long gowns and middle class children wear 34–inch gowns, in the early 20th century, it was more generally thought that a child's health was of more importance than its class.[21] "If the baby's body is restricted about the abdomen, the internal organs will become displaced and cause deformity and suffering all through life...The little baby's long clothing is often made too long and too heavy; and the mother's delight in the long, pretty dresses, and her desire to keep her baby as long as she can, often leads her to keep it too long in long dresses."[22]

As such quotes allude to, unfortunately for many children, a great many mothers were little more than children themselves. In the United States, courting at the age of 14 was perfectly permissible up through the 19th century, and in 1890, 20 million American females were wed at age fourteen.[23] Still, it's an exaggeration to say that most brides were children. The average woman of the 1890s wed at 22 (the 1790s statistic is surprisingly aged—27) and, in general, American women were most properly thought wed if they were in their 20s—though they shouldn't wait until they hit 30, because, as *The Household Magazine* explained, "If a woman is thirty and unmarried, men straightway question for the reason, and then seek no farther [sic.] acquaintance because someone hasn't made the Miss a Mrs. before."[24]

Though some "experts" believed that "premature love robbed the nerve and brain of their natural needs and blighted the organs of sex,"[25] it was generally accepted in the United States that bearing children—even at a relatively young age—did wonders for women. It was alleged that it made females healthier, and prevented the later curse of menopause. Not only was motherhood the "fulfillment of a woman's physiological and moral destiny,"[26] but it was thought that "bearing children tends to keep beauty of form and feature—other things being equal—even increasing it sometimes, and putting old age a long way off."[27]

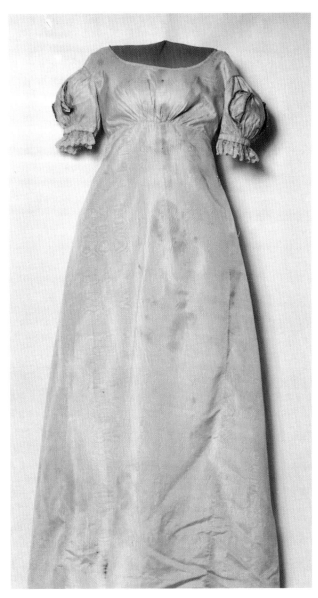

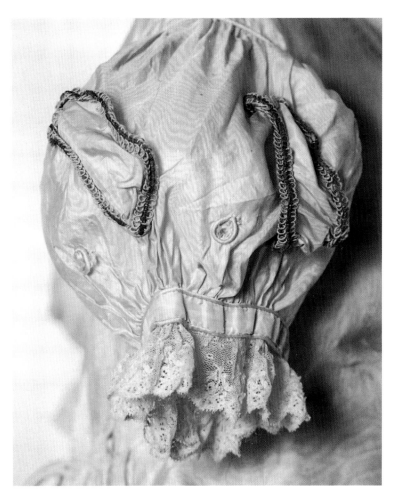

A young misses' evening gown, c.1815–20, cut with a slim skirt, a high-waisted bodice gathered at center front, and cap sleeves trimmed with lace and braid. The hand sewn gown closes in back with one hook and eye at the neck and another at the waist. A fabric drawstring at the back waist further secures the gown. *Courtesy of Vintage Silhouettes.* In current condition $75–$125; in very good condition $600—$1,000.

Nonetheless, this author cannot help but believe that Victorian "prudery" had more to do with the dangers (including fatalities) inherit in childbearing than with anything else. Few doctors could be bothered to deliver babies, leaving the work up to neighbors, family members, and mid–wives—making women personal witnesses to the tragedies associated with childbirth. Meanwhile, as sex education books of the Victorian period warned that "it is better for our daughters that they should not know what awaits them in marriage, 'lest their hearts fail them,'"[28] it was nonetheless considered of great importance to prepare girls for motherhood, even from an early age. "All the way from childhood onward, the wise mother will be installing truths into the minds of her daughters, that will be along the line of preparation for motherhood," the author of *What Every Young Wife Ought To Know* advised. "The early teaching of truth, the early knowledge of self and sex relations, the right estimate of marriage, all these lessons are preparing the way for the later knowledge that precedes motherhood. From the wedding day, the young matron should shape her life to the probable and desired contingency of conception and maternity. Otherwise she had no right or title to wifehood."[29]

And for women living before the legalization of birth control in the 1930s, having children—often one right after the other—was not just a "desired contingency," but a fact of life. "Mother said that she did not know whether she had mentioned the fact that we have another son," one woman wrote in a letter to her sister in 1872. "Such a common occurrence that it is no novelty."[30] Even so, previous to the 'teens, pregnancy required the dreaded "confinement"—a tradition of staying in the house and out of sight of the public when in the last trimester. After all, as *The Household Magazine* so aptly put it, "a modest woman does not needlessly publish her secret."[31]

Unfortunately, even up through the 1920s, a woman's pregnancy was full of myth and folklore—often spread by medical doctors. "The common people often get at truths in a rude way long before the scientists do," one Dr. Holbrook was quoted as saying in the early 1900s. "Many parents tell us their children are strongly influenced by some particular occupation of the mother during pregnancy. So strong is this belief that many mothers are in our time trying to influence the characters of their unborn children by special modes of life, by cultivating music, or art, or science, in order to give the child a love for these pursuits."[32] This notion—though it might sound odd coming from a doctor—might sound possible (even probable) to us today, but in the 19th and early 20th century, the idea was exaggerated. In 1870, for example, a Professor Oswald Fowler asked whether "a pregnant mother's experiences affect the offspring?" His own answer was resounding; "Indeed they do. The eminent Dr. Napheys reports the case of a pregnant lady who saw some grapes, longed intensely for them, and constantly thought of them. During the period of her gestation she was attacked and much alarmed by a turkey–cock. In due time she gave birth to a child having a large cluster of globular tumours growing from the tongue and exactly resembling our common grapes. And on the child's chest there grew a red excrescence exactly resembling a turkey's wattles."[33]

Even after the baby's birth, most of its raising was left up to women—its mother and, if the family was of some means, a nurse or nanny. The father's role was merely to "teach her to live under obedience, and whilst she is unmarried, if she would learn anything, let her ask you, and afterwards her husband."[34] There was some guidance for mothers, however. Women's magazines often gave terse and infrequent tips on child–rearing, how–to books abounded by the late 19th century, and as early as 1842, *Parents Magazine* was being published. Some advice, however, would have been best left unheard. Up until the mid–19th century, for example, the mother's milk was regarded not as milk—but rather as a bleached form of the blood that nourished the child in the womb. And up through the 1860s, the habit of taking drugs to aid nursing was a common practice—even if *Godey's Lady's Book* condemned it by saying "the habit of resorting to tea, coffee, wines, cordials, and various stimulating drinks, under the mistaken notion that they increase the milk and impart strength, is more pernicious, and is ruinous to the health of nurse and child."

In that same issue, *Godey's* quoted a doctor as advising the use of drugs—in particular, opiates—to calm and soothe babies.[35] Carrie Nation, best known for her hatchet–carrying (and using) during her temperance work in the 19th century, claimed that even children were alcoholics in America. In the South, she claimed, everyone—from wee babes to grandparents—drank mint whiskey upon waking up in the morning (much like today's adults drink their "wake up" coffee). Crying babies were routinely given alcohol to soothe them; rum with peppermint added was a common "cure" for childhood measles; and pregnant women were told by doctors to take milk and rum to ensure an easy pregnancy and delivery.[36]

Those who could afford to, however, often rested the fate of their babes not in the hands of doctors and how–to books, but in the hands of nurses. Though as early as the 1740s, wet–nursing was being condemned as the cause of high infant mortality, the practice continued through most of the Victorian era. Nonetheless, by the mid–19th century, wet–nurses were rare—rare enough, that Alice Roosevelt, the high–spirited daughter of President Theodore Roosevelt, spoke of her own experience with a wet–nurse with some embarrassment. "My brother Ted found out...from one of the nurses, doubtless...that after my mother died I had had a wet nurse," she said. "So this horrid little cross–eyed boy of about five would go around to all and sundry exclaiming, 'Sissy had a sweat nurse!'...It was frightfully wounding to the character! I certainly wasn't going to put up with everyone saying, 'The poor little thing.'"[37]

Still, despite much mis–information and dubious practices, by the mid–19th century, the infant mortality rate was on decline—so much so, in fact, that infants were being allowed out in public for more than just their christenings. "The child and its mother are no longer relegated to the woman's apartments as in the past," one man noted in his diary. "The child is shown while still an infant. Parents proudly present the child's nurse. It's as if they were on stage, making a great show of their production."[38]

This 1825 fashion plate illustrates a somewhat similar dress, featuring a gathered bodice set into a skirt whose fullness is gathered in back. The child wears a typically simple muslin dress with short sleeves and a high waist, worn over pantalettes.

### Endnotes:

[1] *Godey's Lady's Book*, 1857, p.169
[2] *The Sunday Sentinel*, March 29, 1914; *Ladies Home Journal*, June 1918
[3] *Children's Costume In England*, p.107
[4] *The Workwoman's Guide*, 1838, p.150
[5] *Woman's Institute of Domestic Arts & Sciences*
[6] *Godey's Lady's Book*, June 1832, p.268
[7] New York City statistics for 1853; Massachusettes statistics for 1850; *Light of Home*, p.166
[8] *Century of Childhood*, p.49–50
[9] *Godey's Lady's Book*, 1857 p.267
[10] ibid, p.362
[11] *The Awakening*, p.17
[12] *The Lady's Economical Assistant*, 1808, p.147
[13] *The Workwoman's Guide*, 1838
[14] *McCall's*, Feb. 1913, p.41
[15] *Art of Dressmaking*, p.105
[16] *What A Young Wife...*, p.144
[17] *McCall's*, Feb. 1913 p.42
[18] *What a Young Wife...*, p.164–170
[19] *Dombey and Son*

[20] *Godey's Lady's Book*, 1857, p.362
[21] *The Workwoman's Guide*, 1840, p. 55
[22] *Home & Health*, p.259
[23] *Fabulous Century*, p.188
[24] *The Household*, Aug. 1874
[25] *Light of Home*, p.21
[26] *Godey's Lady's Book*, Dec. 1860
[27] *Demorests' Monthly Magazine*, June 1887, p.29
[28] *What A Young Wife...*, p.37
[29]. ibid, p.100–01
[30] Susan Huntington Hooker, Aug. 19, 1872; *Light of Home*, p.33
[31] *The Household Magazine*, Ap. 1879
[32] *What A Young Wife...*, p.144
[33] *Everyday Life*, p.170
[34] *Weaker Vessel*, p.149
[35] *Godey's Lady's Book*, Dec.1860
[36] *Vessel of Wrath*, p.101–02
[37] *Mrs. L.*, p.16–18
[38] *History of Private Life*, p.322

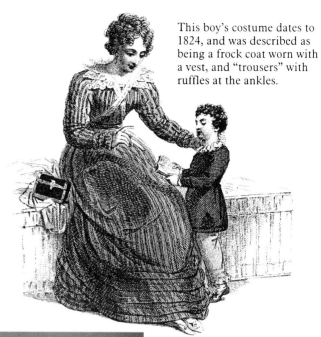

This boy's costume dates to 1824, and was described as being a frock coat worn with a vest, and "trousers" with ruffles at the ankles.

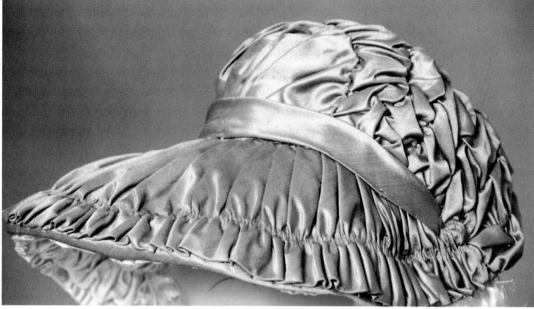

This early 19th century silk bonnet is mounted onto a wire frame and is meticulously ruched. *Courtesy of Vintage Silhouettes.* $250—$400.

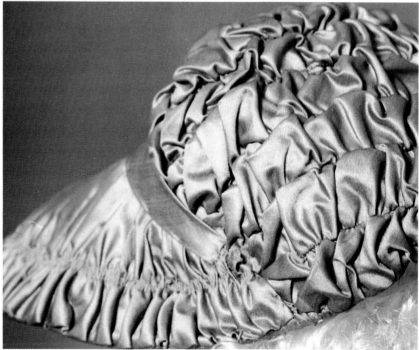

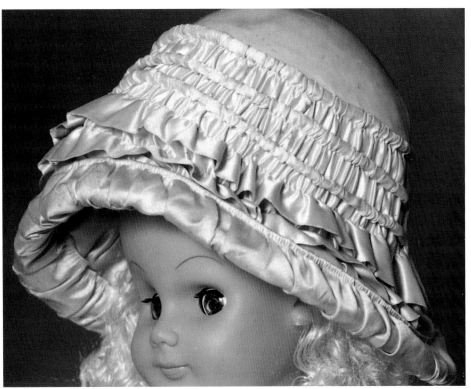

A c.1820s–30s girl's bonnet of cream-colored silk, lined with ruched pink silk and mounted onto a wire frame. *Courtesy of Vintage Silhouettes.* $250—$400.

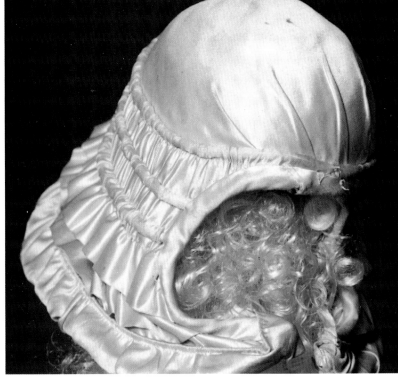

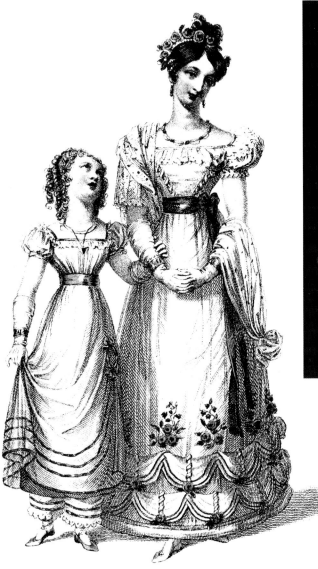

An 1826 fashion plate from *Repository of Arts, Literature, Commerce, Manufactures, Fashions and Politics.* The girl's dress is described as white silk gauze, edged with blue satin and blonde lace. The skirt is trimmed with blue satin pipings, and a blue satin slip is worn beneath the whole, along with white cambric pantalettes.

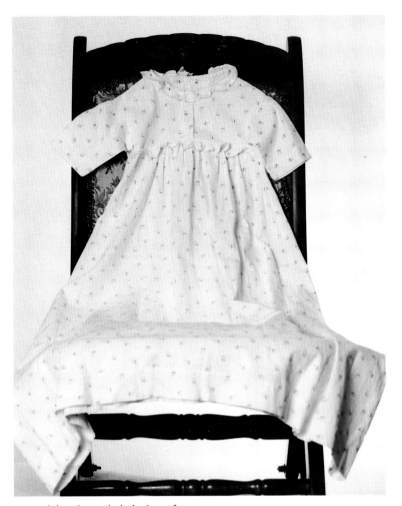

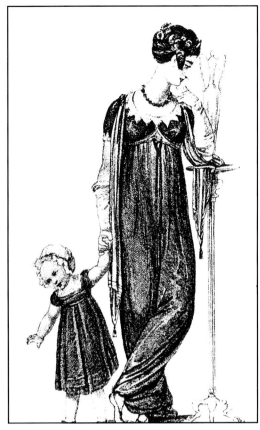

This little girl's dress from an 1809 fashion drawing is of a cut similar to those worn throughout the 19th and early 20th century.

A handsewn baby's dress from the first quarter of 19th century. It is fashioned of a printed cotton and features self–ruffles at the neck and waistline. There is no indication of fasteners in back, indicating that it was originally pinned closed. *Courtesy of Antique Apparel.* $300—$450.

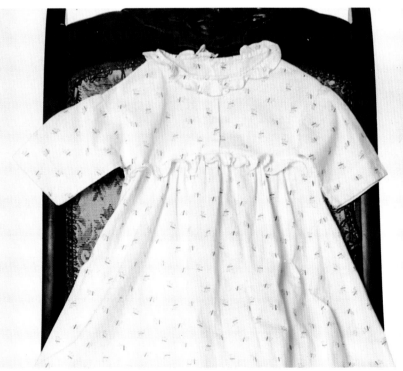

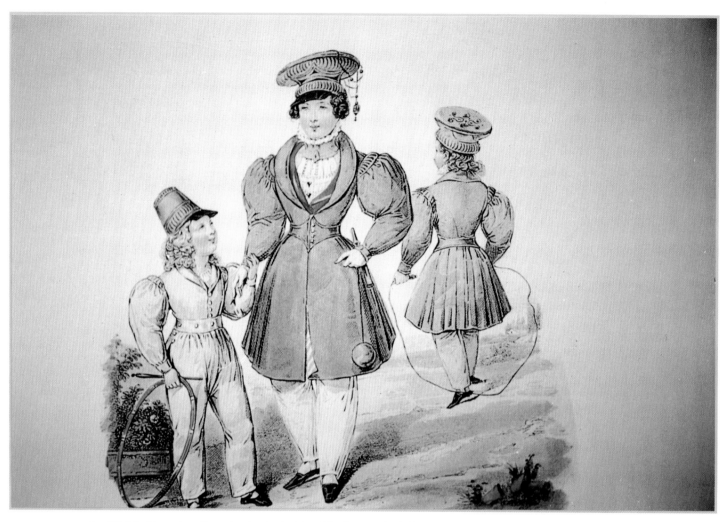

A c.1830 fashion plate featuring boy's clothing. The boy on the left wears a very simple suit of trousers, while the boy at center wears a more elaborate suit consisting of trousers (with straps to slip over the foot), a fussy, lace–trimmed shirt, a vest, and a jacket. Both boys wear the full, puffed sleeves associated with women's fashions of the era. $65—$95.

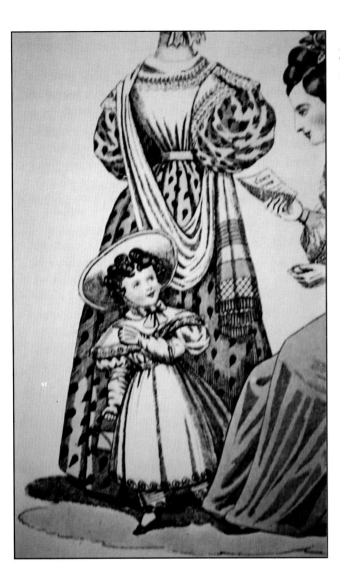

An 1831 fashion plate, showing a girl wearing a dress that varies little from her mother's. $65—$95.

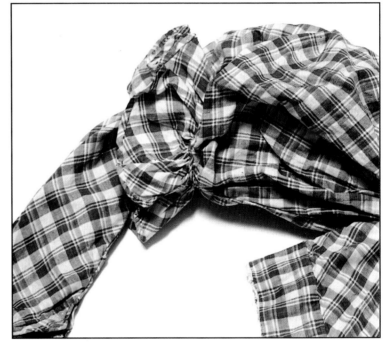

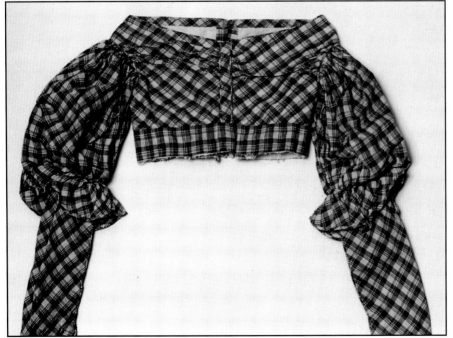

A c.1837–1841 hand sewn baby's bodice of a cotton plaid. The wide neckline is set off by piping and a flange from shoulder to waist in back. Piping is also featured in the armhole seam and on the puffed sleeves. A string with one edge tacked to the inside of the shoulder seam and the other end tacked to the end of each puff, prevents the puffs from falling straight and keeps them full. Hooks and eyes close the bodice in back, while the center front is gathered vertically into a band. *Courtesy of Vintage Silhouettes.* $150—$200.

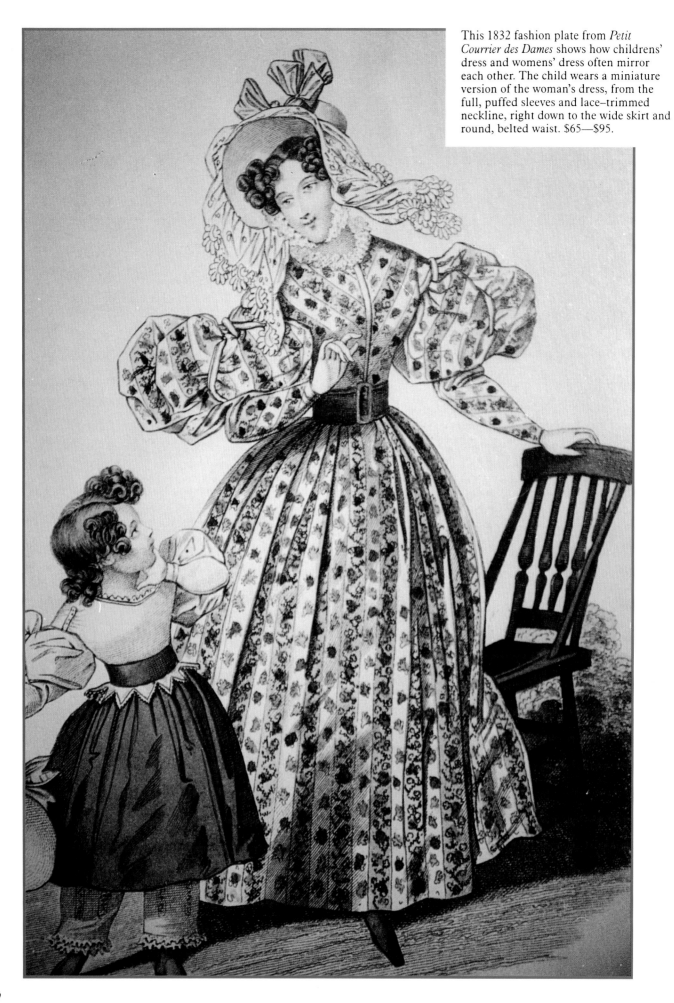

This 1832 fashion plate from *Petit Courrier des Dames* shows how childrens' dress and womens' dress often mirror each other. The child wears a miniature version of the woman's dress, from the full, puffed sleeves and lace–trimmed neckline, right down to the wide skirt and round, belted waist. $65—$95.

# In 'Coats

Fashion magazines rarely mentioned children's clothes in the 18th, 19th, and early 20th centuries; like today's fashion magazines, their focus was on women's styles. However, as early as 1779 *Lady's Magazine* offered a plagiarized version of *Emile* to its readers, and by circa 1814, most fashion magazines mentioned one or two outfits a year for children under six years old. It wasn't until the 1860s that fashions for teenagers were discussed and pictured; at this same time, the first magazines devoted entirely to an audience of children appeared—notably, *The Young Ladies' Journal*. After the 1860s, children's fashions became a regular feature in most fashion magazines, and by the 1880s, some magazines even featured several whole color fashion plates devoted entirely to children's wear.

In the early years of the 19th century, boys were wearing a sort of cross between a man's suit and a jumper, called a "skeleton suit." Charles Dickens described this as "one of those straight blue cloth cases in which small boys used to be confined...fastening him into a very tight jacket, with an ornamental row of buttons over each shoulder and then buttoning his trousers over it so as to give his legs the appearance of being hooked on just under the armpits..."[1] First introduced in the 1790s, and finding its strongest run from about 1800 through the 1830s, the skeleton suit didn't go entirely out of favor until the 1850s. However, up through the 1890s or so, dresses were still the favorite garb for little boys.

"The difficulty of artistically costuming a very tiny boy is one which most mothers have, at some time or other, had ample reason to appreciate," *The Standard Designer* confessed.[2] Indeed, the entire issue of when to breech boys was still hotly debated, and it is startling for most modern readers to find that many fashion magazines, when describing clothing suitable for children, often pointed out that many dresses were "suitable for either boy or girl." There were some distinguishing differences, however. "Little boys' dresses button up the front, those of their sisters fasten in back," *Ladies' Home Journal* emphasized.[3] While girls were expected to rely on others to dress them throughout most of the 19th century, it was expected and desired that little boys should become independent—and learning how to dress themselves early on was important. Another indication that a dress belonged to a little boy and not a little girl was a wide ribbon running crosswise across the body, from one shoulder to the opposite hip; similarly, dresses with a button closure running from one shoulder, crosswise to the hem, were designed for boys.

Nonetheless, while a boy was "still in 'coats," he found himself looking an awful lot like his sister. "For small boys dresses of velvet are very much worn...The ruffled pantalette comes below the dress, and a cloth gaiter keeps the limbs warm..."[4] Still, there were perhaps more important differences between his dress and his sister's. "On a cold and frosty evening," Mrs. Merrifield wrote in her book *Dress As A Fine Art*, "the boys were all dressed in high dresses up to the throat, while the bands which encircled their waists were so loose as merely to keep the dress in its place without confining it; in short, their dress did not offer the slightest restraint on their freedom of movement. It was otherwise with the girls...they were dressed in low dresses, and their shoulders were so bare, that we involuntarily thought of a caterpillar casting its skin...[but] we realized that this was rendered impossible by the tightness of the clothes about the waist...It entirely destroyed their freedom of movement." Merrifield also noted that it was easy to see the girls were corseted, and the boys were not, when they moved to pick up a ball off the floor: "The boys always stoop, while the girls...invariably drop on one knee."[5]

Others, however, argued that while it was perfectly reasonable for girls to be in frilly dresses, it was absurd for boys to dress in the same fashion. "It is bad enough, in all conscience to pervert the mind and character of girls, and render them dressed up in bundles of vanity," wrote the author of *Nursery Book For Young Mothers*, "but boys—boys who are to become men—it is shocking! Of all weaknesses in a man, what is more despicable than an inordinate love of dress, added to an exorbitant desire for admiration of self...? If you make him a peacock now, there is much reason to apprehend that he will never become an eagle."[6]

The aim of most mothers, then, was to find a "little suit so cute that no mother will be able to resist [it], however unwilling she may be to lose her baby in her boy."[7] By the 1860s, this had become a more sensible, adult style. "For little boys hovering between dresses and the first pair of 'pantaloons,'" *Godey's* suggested, "we recommend short trousers or drawers of white linen, and cambric saques of plain colors, pale green, blue, pink, or buff, with a narrow edge of white braid in parallel rows. They should be made low in the neck, very loose, and with

"The careful mother, having an eye to the preservation of pretty frocks, will find it to her advantage to provide her little women with a plentiful supply of aprons." *The Standard Designer*, 1897

short sleeves. A broad belt of patent leather will confine them sufficiently at the waist. For the street, high brown–linen aprons, of saque pattern, are a sufficient protection, the belt to be worn upon the outside, [the] sleeves long."[8] Boys were now wearing button–fly openings—even though grown men still clung to the old style front flaps. Boys also popularized the blazer during this time—before men ever even considered wearing it.

The blazer had been popular wear for boys since the 1850s—and was sometimes worn by boys previous to that time. It was usually called a "short jacket," and was probably only referred to as a blazer after the late 1880s, when the Cambridge Boat Club's members donned adult–sized versions in scarlet red. (The sailors of the English ship *H.M.S. Blazer* claimed that, in fact, the jacket was named after them, but this is unlikely since it appears that the Cambridge boaters scarlet jackets came first.)

For girls, on the other hand, "there is so little difference between the dress of little girls and their mothers', that there is not much to say as to styles for them."[9]

Up through the 1860s, girls dresses frequently had rounded necklines ending at the base of the neck—or, for evening, very scooping necklines, seemingly falling off the shoulders and onto the upper arms. Since circa 1827, waistlines had been in their natural position, and by the 1850s, this style was vastly popular. From the 1840s through the 1860s, such bodices were usually lined with stiff booking muslin, and often had whaleboning inserted into the seams, just like the adult versions. By day, sleeves were long and modest, but by evening—again imitating their mothers' dresses—sleeves were very short and puffed. *Godey's Lady's Book* was one of the few fashion magazines to condemn this style. "There is [a] foolish and pernicious fashion we have also warned mothers to avoid—that of dressing little children in low–necked frocks. Boys are exempted from this display of their fair shoulder at an early age, but little girls are, by the absurd and, we must use plain language, wicked vanity of their mother, often subjected to such an uncomfortable as well as injurious mode of dress, till their forms are permanently injured."[10]

By the 1880s, dress reform had become such a popular subject that whole magazines were devoted to the issue. Though their articles were almost always focused on women's fashions, girls' clothing also invariably came up. In *Dress*, the premiere magazine on dress reform, one issue focused in on "How Shall We Clothe Our Children?" The editors admitted that "this question is...often asked us by intelligent mothers," and that they felt compelled to deal with the issue because there was so little literature on the subject. "In the meantime...the little ones are crying, and many of us know the cause is often lack of proper clothing. The mistake is made not only by the poor and impoverished, but also in the families of the rich and well–to–do...Examine the clothing of almost any child you meet, and you will find, on comparison with your own, that you would be cold with the same weight and amount of clothing...*Keep the extremities warm.* Cover well the arms and legs, and the rest of the body will be comfortable. This, of course, disposes of the cruel, wicked fashion of leaving the knees naked." [11]

By the same token, however, others condemned girl's clothing as being too heavy. The same magazine warned: "Do not allow the girls to wear heavy petticoats pressing down over the hips—the custom is deadly."[12] And while "broderie anglaise" (or eyelet) became an immensely popular material for girls' dresses in the 1860s (perhaps because, as costume expert Doris Langley Moore suggested, with the advent of the hoopskirt layers upon layers of adult women's petticoats were no longer needed—so mothers cut them up and recycled them for their children), fashion magazines were touting: "They are not puppets, made for the display of fine clothes; or Paris dolls to be tricked out in the extravagance of latest fashion...How much happier are the little careless creatures for being decked like so many opera dancers, with velvet cloaks and voluminous ruffles, gaiters that chill their delicate feet and satin bonnets that do not even shield their faces?"[13]

The pleas to and from mothers seemed endless by the 1880s. In the end, it was probably mothers' sympathies that led to more sensible girls' clothing: "Many women who will not embrace radical innovations in dress for themselves will gladly welcome such improvement for their children as will insure for them strong and vigorous maturity," one mother wrote to *Dress*. Another fashionable woman wrote, "Women are thinking upon the subject of rational dress; and although many of us, who have always been accustomed to our tightly laced corsets and very little physical exercise, would find it difficult, if not impossible, to adopt radical changes in our own costumes, we are ready and anxious for it for our girls."[14]

Nonetheless, in the midst of all this were girls wearing hoopskirts and bustles. Though some boys apparently did wear hoopskirts for special occasions only, many girls wore them

---

*What A Little Girl Should Be Taught*

To cook plain, wholesome food.
To make her own clothes.
To be neat and orderly, beginning with the care of her own person and room.
That she should learn well the arts of housekeeping and home-making before trying to make a home of her own.
That she should exercise quiet reserve in the presence of boys and men.
That all cheap talk is unbecoming.
That loose jokes about 'beaux' and 'lovers' are improper.
That modesty is a priceless treasure, and will prove her surest protector.

That her brothers are better escorts than most other young men.
That her mother is her best companion and counselor.
That her dress should be plain, and should not be the chief subject of her thoughts or conversation.
That she should wear only such styles of clothing as will cover her person modestly.
That it is better to be useful than ornamental.
That there will be time enough to learn fancy work after she has learned to darn stockings.
That the old rule, 'A place for everything and everything in its place,' is a good one.
That she should dress for health and comfort as well as for appearance. *Home & Health, 1907*

*What A Little Boy Should Be Taught*

To be strong and brave—to be a little man.
To shun evil companions.
To respect gray hairs.
To be gentle.
To be courteous.
To be prompt.
To be industrious.
To be truthful.
To be honest.
To seek companionship of his sisters in preference to any other
    girls.
To honor his father and his mother.

To be temperate.
To discard profanity.
To be thoughtful and attentive.
To keep himself pure.
To be his sister's protector
To refuse to listen to vulgar jokes or stories.
To use common tools skillfully.
To care for his own room
To do all kinds of housework.
To earn money and to take care of it.
To be neat and orderly in his habits and appearance.
To be self–reliant.
To be his father's partner. *Home & Health, 1907*

everyday. In the world of women's fashions, hoopskirts (or crinolines, as they were sometimes called) were touted as offering much freedom to women who had previously wore many layers of petticoats to hold out their skirts. As anyone who has ever worn several layers of petticoats knows, they have a tendency to wrap around the legs, making walking difficult. And so, little girls—whether rich or poor—often wore hoops for the freedom they gave. Some hoops were fashioned at home with cane, but many were made of wire and were bought inexpensively from ready–to–wear sources. Nonetheless, hoops managed to still reign in girls, since they made rambunctious play impossible. One mother, writing to a magazine editor in 1858, asked if there was any way for her daughter to avoid embarrassment when she climbed, jumped, and partook in other childhood activities. The editor's reply was simple; the girl should "not attempt the climbing of stiles in a crinoline for the task is impossible. And if she suffers much from the comments of vulgar little boys it would be better, in a high wind, to remain indoors."[15]

With the thanks of many little girls, by 1870 hoops were going out of fashion—but in their place, the bustle protruded. Unlike hoops, bustles were primarily reserved for special occasion wear, with day dresses having little puffs and folds of fabric to simulate the look of a bustle by day. Though bustles were far less embarrassing and confining than hoops, they did, nonetheless, hinder activity. Still, most girls seem to have enjoyed them. "My sister and me had black velvet frocks for the occasion, and I were as proud as a peacock 'cos I had a proper little bustle at the back," Sybil Marshall wrote of attending a christening. "It were made like a little square pincushion about nine inches long and four or five inches wide, and I tied it round my waist afore putting my frock on."[16] Marshall was speaking of the small, cushion bustle, worn when

the bustle style was dying out. In the 1870s and through much of the 1880s, the bustle was a cage–like contraption, much like hoops, but with all the fullness at the rear. And not all little girls found them to be such pleasant things. Alice Roosevelt recalled that after her mother died, she went almost immediately to live with her Aunt Bye, and stayed with her until 1887, when her father remarried. "One of my earliest memories," she said, "is of seeing her bustle hanging in her bedroom in New York. Up to that point, I always considered it an integral part of her anatomy. I was absolutely horrified when I saw it as a separate entity and thought it had been chopped off her by force."[17]

## Endnotes:

[1] *Sketches by Boz*
[2] *Standard Designer*, April 1897
[3] *Ladies Home Journal*, Mar. 1895
[4] *Peterson's Magazine*, 1858
[5] *Dress As A Fine Art*, p.99
[6] *Nusury Book for Young Mothers*, Mrs. Tuthill
[7] *New York Times*, May 7, 1892
[8] *Godey's Lady's Book*, 1860
[9] *Godey's Lady's Book*, Mar., 1860
[10] *Godey's Lady's Book,* 1851
[11] *Dress*, Nov, 1887, p.278–9
[12] ibid, p.282
[13] Sarah J. Hale, *Godey's Lady's Book*, Mar. 1851
[14] *Dress*, Oct.1880
[15] *History of Underclothes*, p.155
[16] *Welcome Sweet Babe*, p.93
[17] *Mrs. L*, p.22

Little Fannie wears a hat
Like her ancient Grannie;
Tommy's hoop was (think of that!)
Given him by Fanny." *Kate Greenaway*

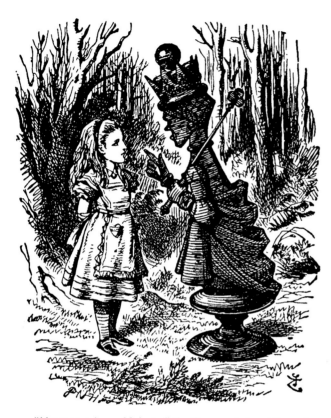

"Always say 'your Majesty,'" the Queen advises Alice, who dons striped stockings, a simple dress, a pinafore, and a simple band in her hair.

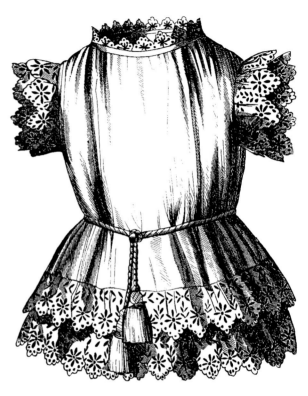

*Godey's Ladies' Book* described this dress from the late 1850s as suitable for girls' six to ten years old. Made of white muslin trimmed with either lace or embroidery, the editor noted that the garment was "light, elegant, and extremely convenient."

### Adventures In Aliceland

In July of 1862, when family friend Reverend Charles Lutwidge Dodgson visited the Liddell family, plucky little Alice Liddell prompted as she often did: "Tell us a story, please." When the Reverend complied and completed an exhaustive narrative about Alice herself, Alice put her hand in his and smiled: "Oh, I wish you would write out Alice's adventures for me." [1]

What resulted was *Alice's Adventures In Wonderland*, first published in 1865 under the Reverend's pen name, Lewis Carrol. With illustrations by Sir John Tenniel, the book found not only literary success, but also influenced the way the way little girls dressed. Beginning in France, and with the publishing of Alice's continued adventures (*Through The Looking Glass*) mothers everywhere turned their daughters into real-life copies of the Reverend's adventuresome heroine. However, unlike some other children's book authors and illustra-

tors that influenced fashion (like Kate Greenaway), the Reverend nor Sir Tenniel actually created new fashions—but they did make massively popular a fledgling style originally reserved for children with aesthetic or transcendentally–minded parents.

Pinafores, for example, had been worn for decades—but combined with the simple Alice dress (not plush or extravagant as many fashionable girl's clothes were), and a new look had been created. Likewise, the "Alice band," or simple ribbon headband worn in unfettered, essentially naturally–styled hair, was a revolutionary idea in fashionable circles. Only Alice's horizontally striped stockings were known in fashionable circles—and in fact, Alice herself did not wear them until the second book...the only instance where the heroine endorsed fashionable attire.

[1.] *Lewis Carroll And His World*, p.5

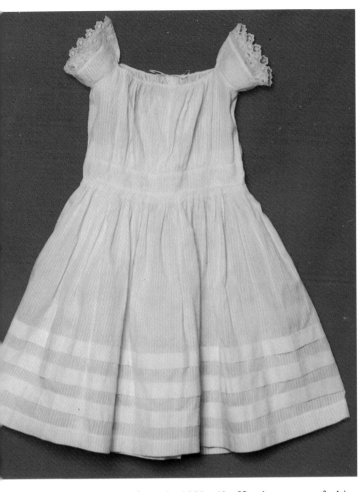

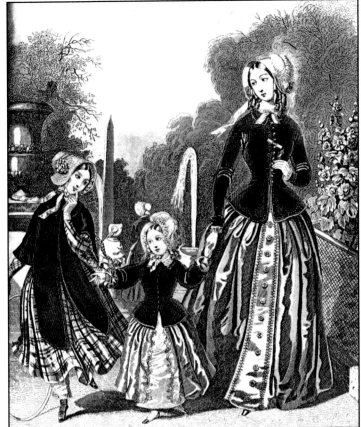

A typical baby's dress from the 1850s–60s. Hand sewn out of white cotton, it features a wide neckline that can be adjusted by a dainty cotton drawstring in back. An additional four buttons close the dress. The bodice is gathered into the waistband, while the skirt is gauged into it. *Courtesy of Mother & Daughter Vintage.* $98—$125.

*The Ladies' National Magazine* boasted that these were the "prettiest costumes ever presented to the American public." The girl on the right wears a dress "of the fashionable plaid, made high in the neck, with tight sleeves. A velvet cardinal [cloak] completes the costume. The bonnet is plainly trimmed with no ornament but a rosette." The younger girl wears a silk dress trimmed with embroidery; her cloak is described as loose–sleeved, and "turned up and puffed at the wrist." Her bonnet is white silk, trimmed with two plumes.

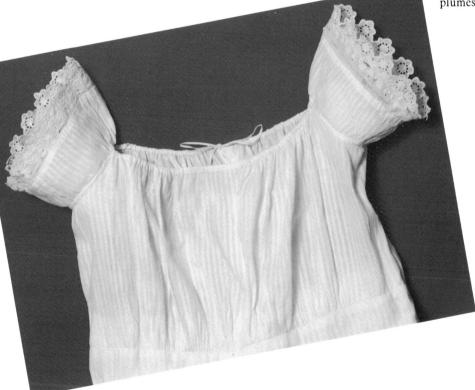

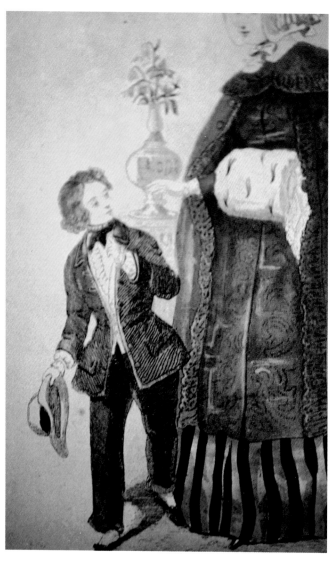

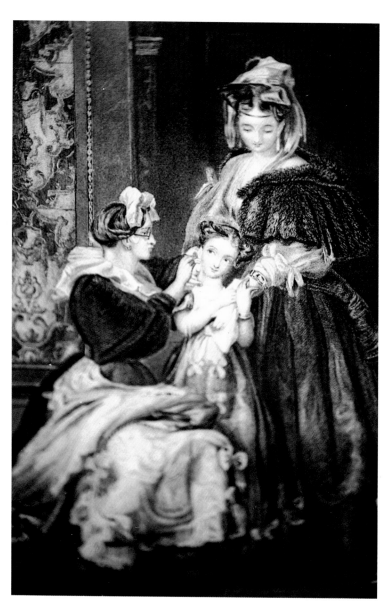

The description for this 1845 fashion plate insists that "the costume of the boy is that most fashionable for lads in Paris!" It features trousers, worn with a white ruffled shirt, tie, and a peplumed jacket reminiscent of 18th century fashions. $45—$75.

An engraving that accompanied the article "The First Ear-Ring," by the editor of *Godey's Lady's Book*, Sarah J. Hale. In the Victorian era, little girls often had their ears pierced. $15—$25.

An 1857 *Godey's Lady's Book* pattern for a jacket for a boy five or six years old, to be made "of velvet...with buttons for ornaments. Velvet is a very suitable material for this charming jacket, which has the advantage of being not only beautiful, but comfortable and healthy. Too many of the jackets, made for little boys, are too open in front, in consequence of which the wearers catch colds on the chest, which often injure their lungs permanently." The boy also wears a hooped skirt.

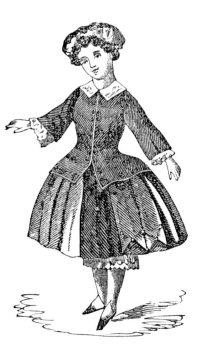

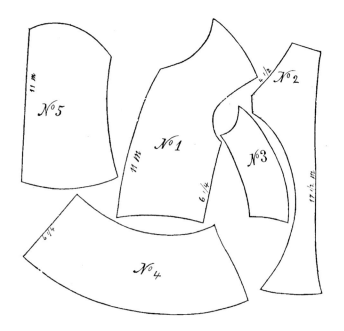

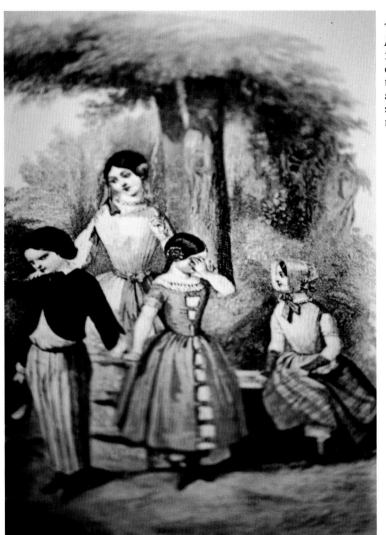

This fashion plate from the May 1849 issue of *Godey's Lady's Book* shows a boy wearing typical attire of the late 1840s—early 50s: a jacket with a rounded front, and loose trousers. The eldest girl wears a "dinner dress" of white with embroidered trim. The girl center front wears a white lawn dress worn under a pink lawn over–dress, while the girl far right wear a coarse straw bonnet lined and trimmed in blue silk, with a simple muslin bodice and silk skirt. $65—$95.

A dress for a boy six or seven years old, from 1857. *Godey's Lady's Book* claimed that with the help of their cutting diagram, "any mother, who has skill in cutting out clothes for her little ones, can make such a [garment] for her son."

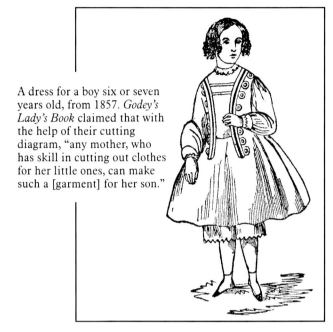

The April 1856 issue of *Godey's Lady's Book* featured these children's costumes, based upon designs by Madame Demorest, the famous dressmaker, fashion magazine publisher, and sewing pattern innovator. The dress is for a girl eight to ten years old and is made of "brilliant lilac." It is "fitted close to the form, with a lace chemisette extending over the shoulders...The skirt is composed of three flounces." The flounces and sleeve caps are scalloped with pinking, "a style of trimming now very much in vogue." The boy's bodice "is gathered into box plaits [pleats] set on a skirt with only a slight fullness, and fastening in front, with buttons and loops. The sleeves are quite full, gathered into a band just below the elbow; another short sleeve or cap is scalloped and gathered up in front."

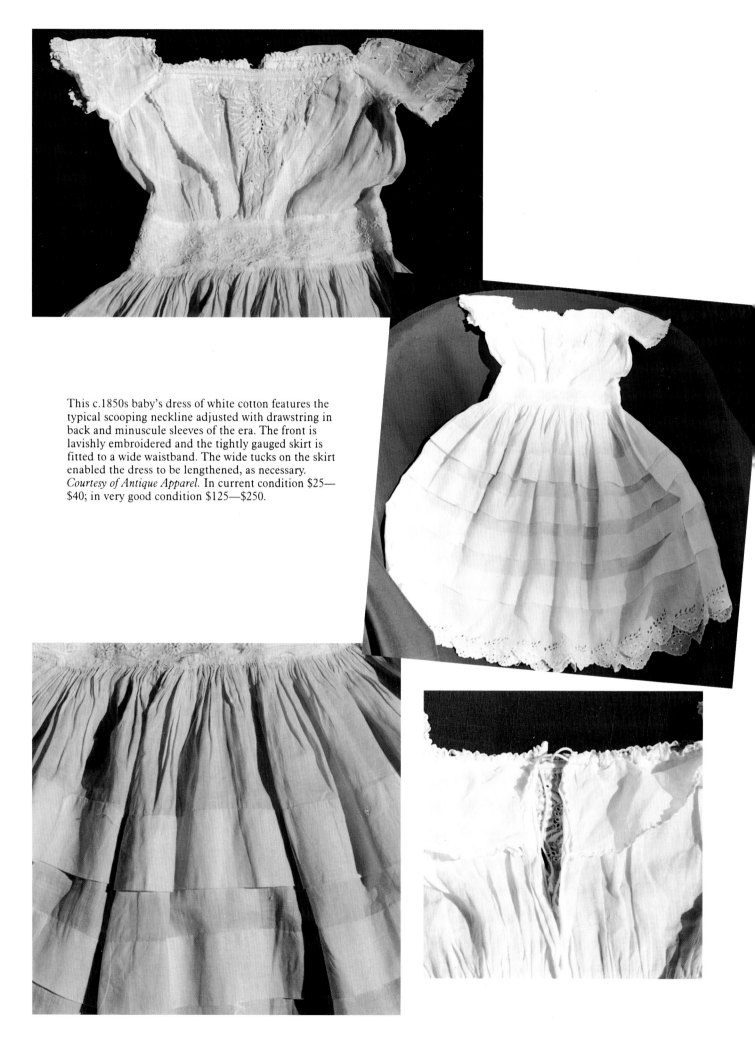

This c.1850s baby's dress of white cotton features the typical scooping neckline adjusted with drawstring in back and minuscule sleeves of the era. The front is lavishly embroidered and the tightly gauged skirt is fitted to a wide waistband. The wide tucks on the skirt enabled the dress to be lengthened, as necessary. *Courtesy of Antique Apparel.* In current condition $25—$40; in very good condition $125—$250.

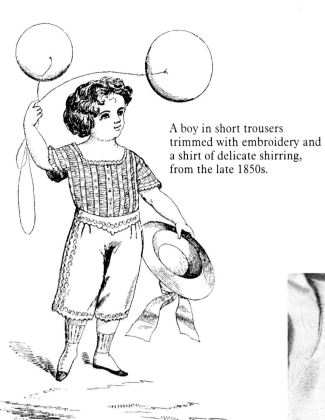

A boy in short trousers trimmed with embroidery and a shirt of delicate shirring, from the late 1850s.

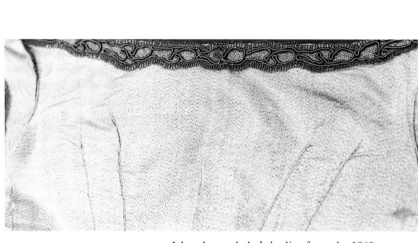

A hand sewn baby's bodice from the 1860s, fashioned out of emerald green changeable silk. The neckline is typically wide and trimmed with braid. The scalloped sleeves and peplum also feature braid trim. Hooks and eyes close the garment in front. *Courtesy of Vintage Silhouettes.* $120—$275.

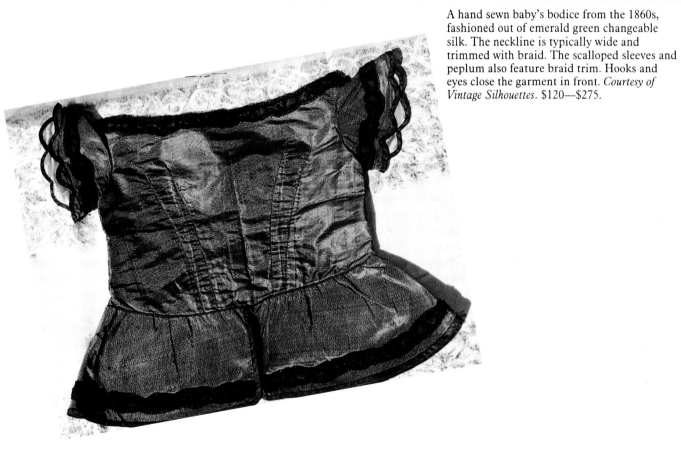

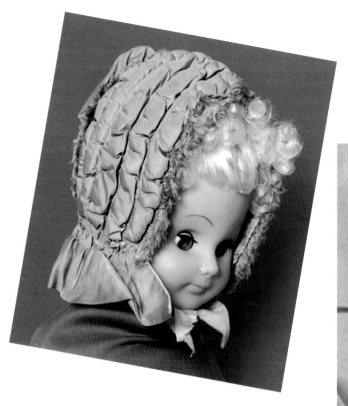

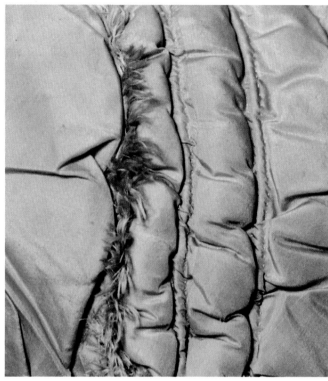

A c.1863–65 grey silk girl's bonnet with puffing and shirring. *Courtesy of Pam Coghan.* $50—$95.

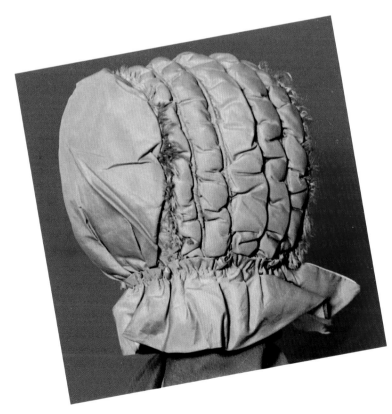

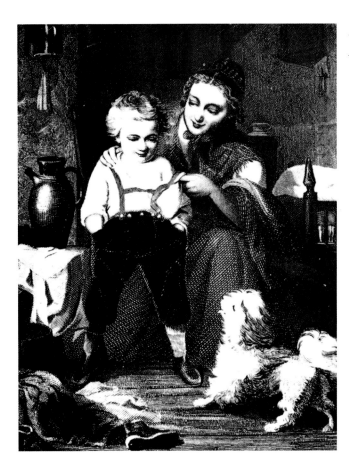

This illustration, which appeared in an 1860 issue of *Peterson's Magazine*, aptly illustrates the ritual of breeching.

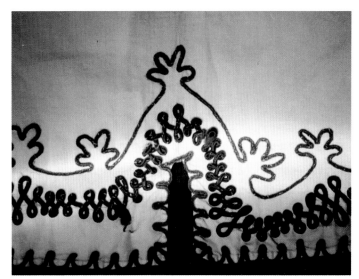

A c.1863–66, hand sewn bolero of cotton with hunter green braid trim. *Courtesy of Antique Apparel.* $45—$85.

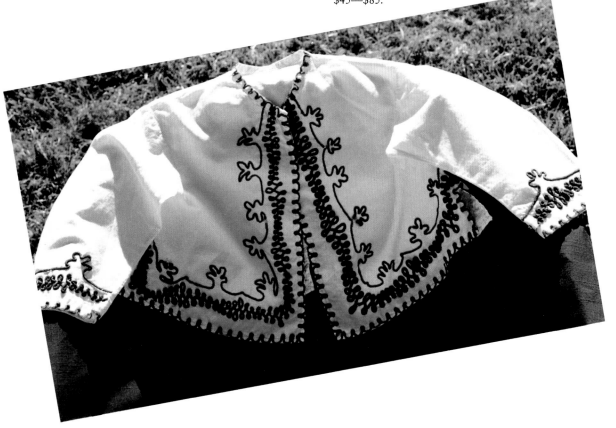

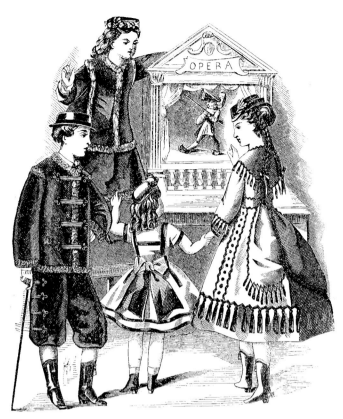

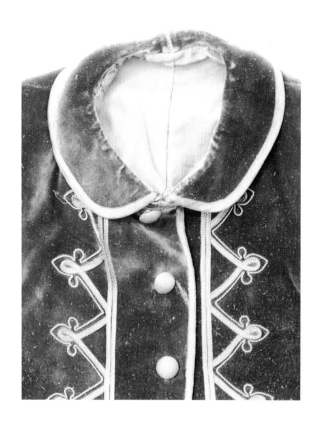

A charming 1868 fashion plate of children's fashions. The boy is described as wearing "short trousers and long jacket...both of black velvet edged with fur, and trimmed with black braid," while the girl standing beside the puppet stage wears a brown velveteen dress edged with Chinchilla. The littlest girl, center front, wears a white mohair dress trimmed with light blue silk, and the girl standing far right wears a dress entirely of blue silk, the skirt, bodice, and sash "all heavily trimmed with a knotted fringe of a shade darker than the dress."

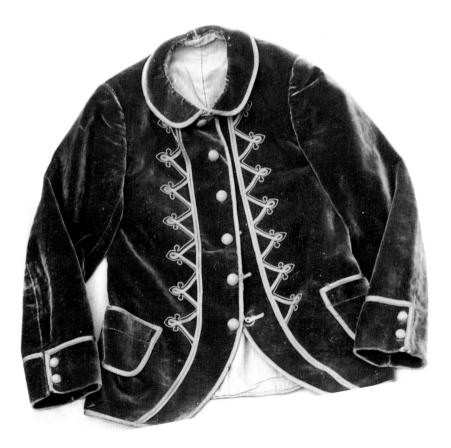

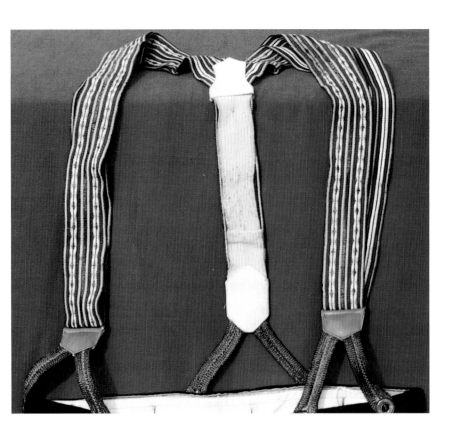

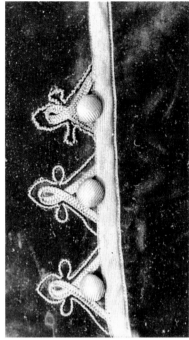

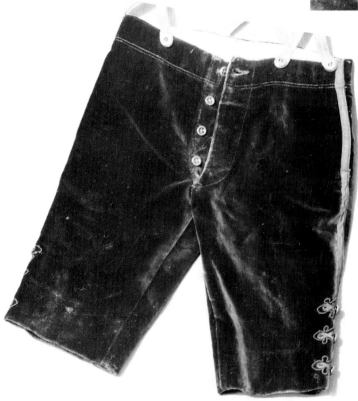

**Opposite page and this page:** This c.1860s boy's suit is made of silk velvet, the knickers are trimmed at their hem with self–covered buttons, binding, and embroidery and were worn with these green and white striped suspenders. The jacket is also trimmed with the same buttons, braid, and binding. *Courtesy of Antique Apparel.* $125—$300.

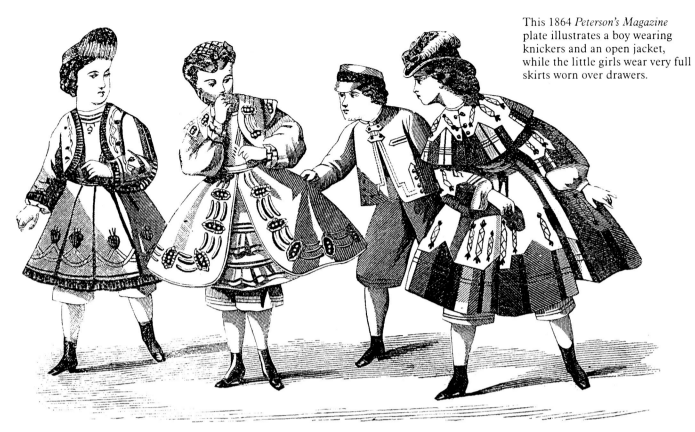

This 1864 *Peterson's Magazine* plate illustrates a boy wearing knickers and an open jacket, while the little girls wear very full skirts worn over drawers.

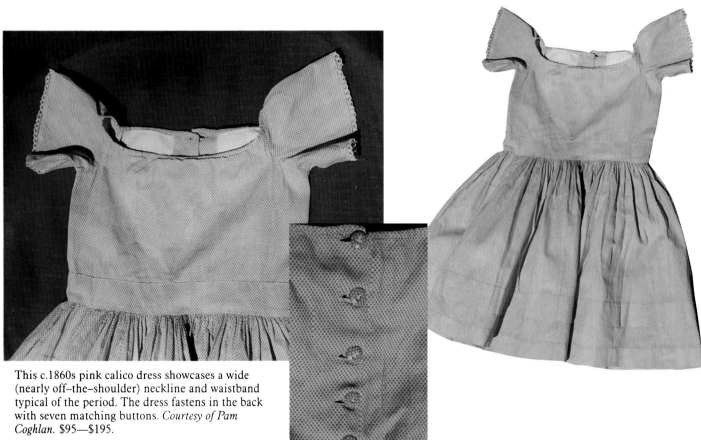

This c.1860s pink calico dress showcases a wide (nearly off–the–shoulder) neckline and waistband typical of the period. The dress fastens in the back with seven matching buttons. *Courtesy of Pam Coghlan.* $95—$195.

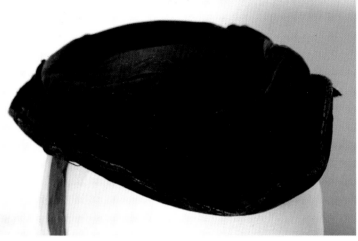

This girl's hat, c.1867–73, is fashioned out of brown and sapphire blue velvet on a wire frame. It has an under the chin tie. *Courtesy of Antique Apparel.* $35—$50.

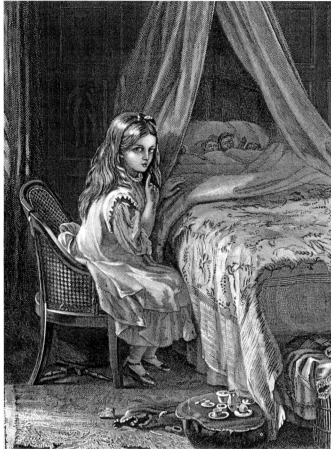

This engraving, titled "The Anxious Mother," appeared in the January 1868 issue of *Peterson's Magazine*. The young girl pictured wears a pinafore, shoes, and ribbon head band in *Alice In Wonderland* style.

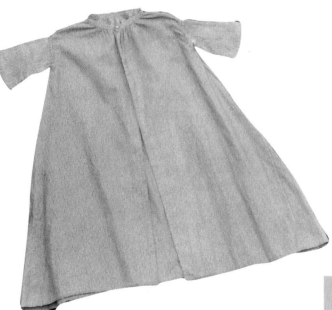

A c.1860s pink and white cotton print apron. A pretty, but utilitarian garment, the apron features sleeves of the most practical length, and is open in back, except for a single pink and white button. The entire garment (including the sleeves) is lined with the same cotton print, so that no seam allowances show. *Courtesy of Cat's Pajamas.* $65—$125.

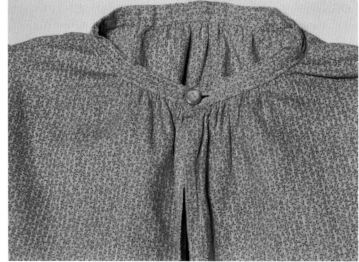

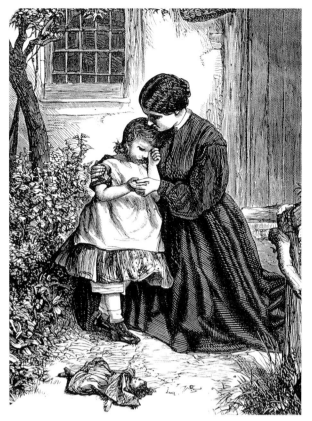

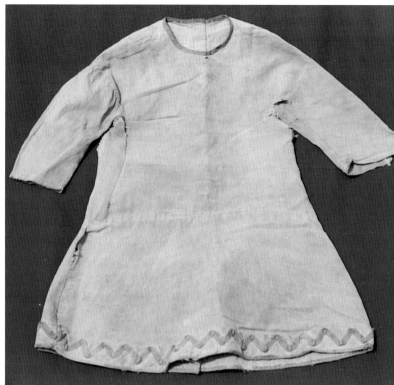

A young girl clad in a practical pinafore, from an 1868 engraving.

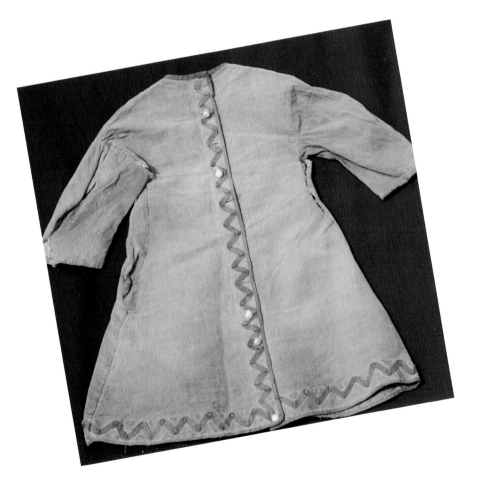

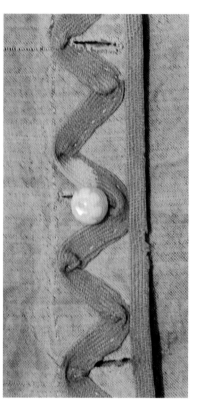

This c.1867–69 boy's dress of cotton is trimmed with what was once red braid and decorative buttons running down the back. *Courtesy of Antique Apparel.* In current condition $15—$30; in very good condition $65—$95.

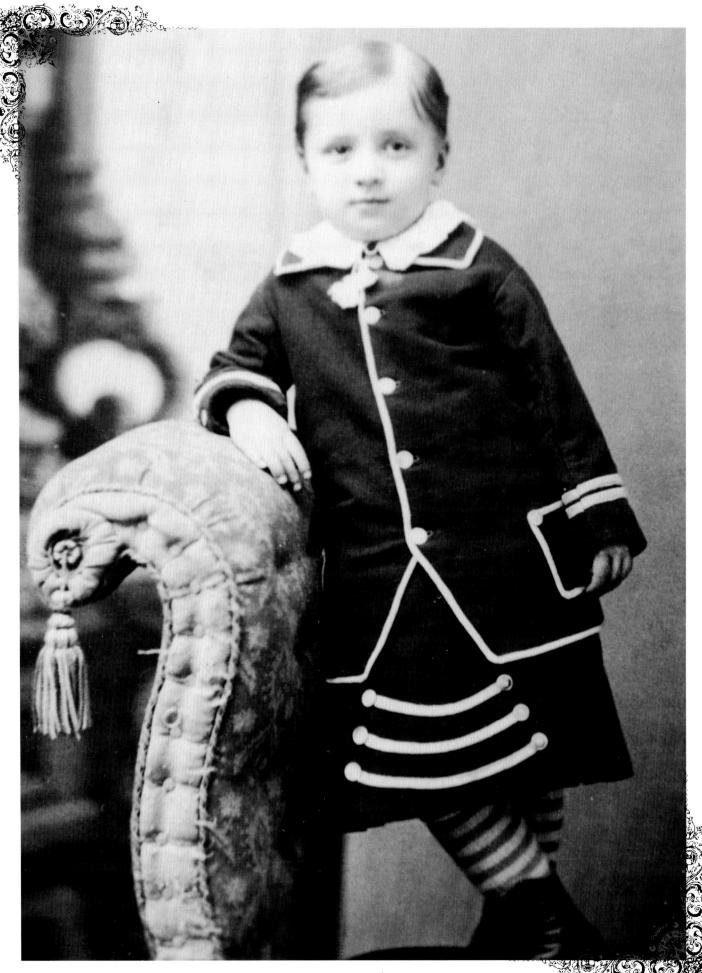

A fashionably dressed boy of the 1860s.

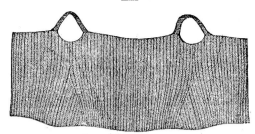

# KNITTED JACKET FOR CHILDREN.

### BY MRS. JANE WEAVER.

MATERIALS.—¼ lb. of No. 6 three-thread knitting cotton, and 2 pins, No. 15.—Cast on 64 stitches, slip the first stitch of every row; the whole is done in plain knitting. Knit 92 rows. 93rd row: Cast off 6 stitches, knit the remainder. 94th row: Plain. 95th row: Cast off 2 stitches, knit the remainder. 96th row: Plain. 97th row: Cast off 2 stitches, knit the remainder. 98th row: Plain. 99th row: Slip 1, knit 2 together, knit the remainder plain. 100th row: Plain, repeat the last 2 rows 6 times more, knit 10 plain rows, then knit only 33 stitches, turn back and knit to the end, next row knit only 32 stitches, then knit to the end. Knit 2 stitches less in every alternate row till only 2 remain; this is to form a gore; then knit the whole number of stitches for 11 rows, then make a stitch at the beginning of every alternate row till 7 increasings are made, knit a plain row after the one with the last increase, then cast on 6 stitches, * knit 12 rows, decrease 1 stitch at the top, repeat from * 5 times more, knit 28 rows, * then increase 1 stitch at the top, knit 12 rows, repeat from * 5 times more, then repeat from the 93rd row till the 6 stitches are cast on, knit 92 plain rows, and cast off. These jackets are much approved for children, as they combine the necessary support with great elasticity, but the knitting must be tightly done to prevent its being too elastic; the shoulder-straps are generally made of tape, but if knitting is preferred, cast on 5 stitches, slip 1, seam 1, knit 1, seam 1, knit 1. Every row is alike. Continue this till you have the length you require for the shoulder-strap. The size given is for a child about three years old, but the same rule may be applied for larger jackets by adding a few more stitches in the casting on, and knitting a few more rows in the width. Few articles are more useful than this.

In 1864 *Peterson's Magazine* offered knitting instructions for this "jacket"—intended to be worn as a piece of underclothing.

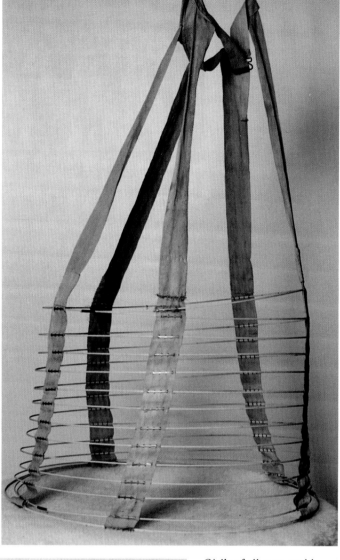

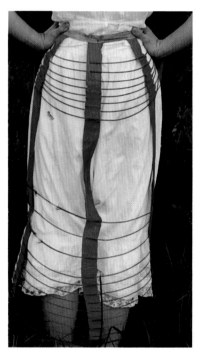

These girl's hoops from the 1860s are metal with unusual, brightly colored tapes. *Courtesy of Antique Apparel.* $95—$125.

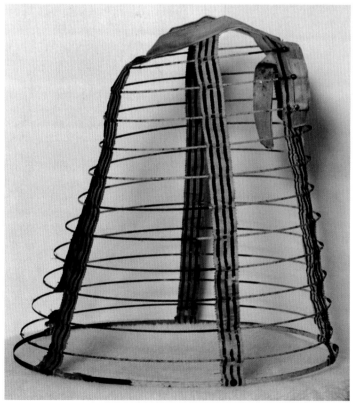

Girl's of all ages could wear hoops—even some boys wore them on very special occasions. Shown here are two typical metal hoops from the 1860s; the smaller of the two features 12 steels and measures a mere 17.5 inches long from waistband to lower steel, and measures 51 inches around the base. The hoops made up of only 14 steels measure 30.5 inches from waistband to lower hoop, and 54 inches around the base. *Courtesy of Vintage Silhouettes.* $110—$135 (12 steels); $100—$130 (14 steels).

*58*

# School Days

"School frocks are now an interesting subject to mothers and daughters," *The Delineator* suggested in the early 1900s. "While practical qualities are to be considered in the selection of these garments, they need not be fashioned with too great severity."[1] Surprisingly, however, while school garments were much the talk in women's magazines that devoted space to children's clothing, in 1900, the literacy rate in the United States was just over 10%, and only 95,000 citizens had graduated from high school.[2] Over 1,700,000 American children under the age of sixteen worked either in factories or in fields. In 1907, the government "remedied" the cruel working conditions such children labored under by minimizing the work week to 66 hours, and by prohibiting night–time work.[3] Looking at even more appalling statistics from the 19th century, early 20th century American children were well off—even without government changes.

About 1.7 million American children under the age of fifteen worked in mines and tobacco fields for as little as 25¢ a day in the 19th century. This was rarely considered improper, and the motto of the era was often cited as being: "The factories need the children and the children need the factories."[4] Truly, the old ideas of children as miniature adults were still shining through. "Cigar–making in the tenement houses goes on, though the fact is often denied," one writer reported in the 1880s. "In cellars and basements boys ten and twelve brine, sweeten, and prepare the tobacco preliminary to stemming. Others of the same age keep the knives of the cutting machines clean by means of sponges dipped in rum...In another workshop children from eight to ten cut the feathers from cock–tails. For ten hours daily they bend over their work...Eight thousand children make envelopes at three and a half cents a thousand. They gum, separate and sort...In [another] factory two hundred children under fifteen are employed spinning, winding and twisting flax; [many] are lacking fingers..."[5] But many people considered such work a blessing because it kept children off the streets. "Little girls are numerous among the street venders," social reformer James McCabe wrote in 1872. "They sell matches, tooth–picks, cigars, newspapers, songs and flowers. The flower girls are hideous little creatures, but the wares are beautiful and command a ready sale."[6] Young street workers were not only exposed to the extremities of the weather, but also to the increasingly evil practices of pimps.

All of this under consideration, it is not surprising to find that the school system as we know it did not come to the United States until a mere 72 years before McCabe wrote. Created by an English Quaker named Joseph Lancaster, an American school system was first founded in 1800. Public schools were by no means cherished by parents, however. Even Louisa May Alcott's father, a noted writer of the period, said that "much systematic instruction is repulsive to the habits and feelings of infancy."[7] Indeed, in the 19th century, the idea of organized schooling was hotly debated.

These early schools, while focusing in the three Rs, were also a means of teaching Christianity and flag worship. "Every morning sees the flag carried to the principal's desk and all the little ones, rising at the stroke of the bell, say with one voice, 'We turn to our flag as the sunflower turns to the sun!' One bell, and every brown right first is raised to the brow, as in military salute: 'We give our heads!' Another stroke, and the grimy little hands are laid on as many hearts: 'And our heart!' Then with a shout that can be heard around the corner: '—to our country! One country, one language, one flag!'" one observer noted.[8]

A boy photographed in the 1870s.

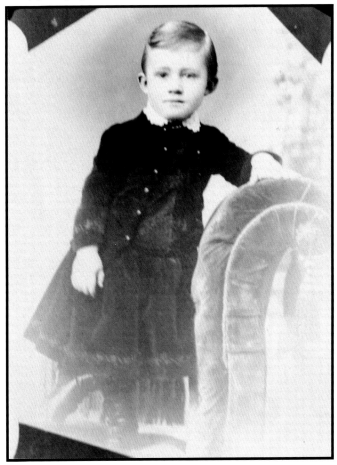

Another important aspect of early education was that of morals and etiquette. Many early American schools echoed the very first childrearing book ever written: *Manners for Children*, originally published in 1530. Cherished by generations long after it premiered, this volume instructed parents and teachers in "the best ways" of teaching children basic societal rules. (One section of *Manners*, for example, pointed out that laughing for no reason "can happen. Politeness then requires you to state the reason for your hilarity. If you cannot do so, you must think of some pretext, lest one of the company think you are laughing at them." Other sections pointed out that "when seated, you must not use of stick or cane to write on the ground or to draw pictures. To do so indicates that you are a dreamer or an ill–bred individual."[9]).

"Under the old system of instruction in this country," *The Delineator* observed in the early 20th century, "education was looked upon as a sort of mental medicine for the child and, like all medicine, was thought to be disagreeable. In the giving of old–time medicine, pleasantness was not considered; and if medicine was needed, it was given in nauseating draughts or huge boluses. Education was needed and consequently it also was given in bitter draughts or boluses. If the child wouldn't take it, he was whipped into swallowing it...The energies of doctor, schoolmaster, parent, were devoted to making the child submissive—to making him swallow the dose."[10] This "old–time schooling," however, was already beginning to change by the 1860s, when the first kindergartens (or "children's gardens") were formed. By the early 1900s, morals, etiquette, and patriotism were often the last things to be taught to children. Instead, as Americans broached the 20th century, such dictates were left to parents—and to boarding schools.

Boarding schools were an accepted way for children to receive their education in the 19th century, but girls' boarding schools were anything but regulated. While some fine schools did exist for girls, a number of shoddy schools marred the image of 19th century girls' boarding schools forever. Victorian novels are littered with accounts of schools where girls

*Greenawismes*

"No one has given us such clear-eyed, soft-faced happy-hearted childhood, or so poetically 'apprehended' the coy reticences, the simplicities, and the small solemnities of little people," said writer Austin Dobson upon seeing artist Kate Greenaway's work at a London gallery. "[And] the old-world costume in which she usually elects to clothe her characters lends an arch piquancy of contrast to their innocent rites and ceremonies."[1]

Though Kate Greenaway was an artist of the late 19th century, she was famous for depicting children in miniature adult costumes of the 1790s; her representation was fairly accurate, and many found the fashions preferable to the more elaborate styles of the 1880s and 1890s. A multitude of mothers copiously copied Greenaway's "new" children's fashions, considering them aesthetically superior.

Dress reform journals were especially quick to pick up on the trend, and early on praised it for its simplicity and beauty. "Picturesque poke bonnets, with high, standing ends and loops in the back, and a wreath of tiny flowers across the front of the crown, are worn by little girls, with quaint costumes en suite,"[2] the editors of *Dress* wrote in 1888 when Greenaway's work first appeared. The look was thought so unique it was dubbed by *La Vie de Paris* as "the graceful mode of Greenawisme."[3]

But it wasn't long before the "charming" Greenawismes were hotly debated. "Opinions remain divided as to the long skirts worn by the babies painted by Kate Greenaway. While some mamas delight in the comical look which long skirts give their little ones, others consider that nothing is more absurd and inconvenient for them than such an imitation of 'grown–up' gowns, and that a little child is not made to be dressed up like a doll for our amusement,"[4] *The Young Ladies' Journal* insisted in 1893.

Perhaps no one, however, published more anti-Greenawismes than Emmeline Raymond, editor and creator of *La Mode Illustrée*. She questioned her faithful readers whether a child dressed in Greenaway costumes was a "little girl or a dwarf,—one hesitates before venturing an opinion."[5]

She ridiculed the style as "eccentric, ungainly, uncomfortable" and described it as having "trailing skirts ruffled at the hem, short–waisted bodices with tucked yolks flanked by ruching, or large shawl collars, crossed and ending in two tall pleated streamers. Sash of draped fabric or ribbon, placed barely under the arms and tied in a bow in back with long tails...Immense hat in the form of a bonnet, with embroidery or lace all around falling over the eyes and forming a curtain. Often the little face, so pleasing to see, disappears under this voluminous headdress, hardly a desirable accessory, and can barely be made out. Thus decked out, the child takes on a bizarre appearance...it's nothing more than a dreary caricature of a creature...Ladies, believe us...Keep Kate Greenaway in her albums..." The style, she insisted, "made veritable caricatures of children."[6]

Whatever the world felt about the fashion, however, Greenaway herself isn't on record as defending it before her untimely death in 1901 at the age of 39. She was not a fashion designer, after all—but an artist. Still, she did write to a friend about what she considered to be an amusing incident:

The lady who has just left me has been staying in the country and has been to see her cousins. I asked if they were growing up as pretty as they promised. 'Yes,' she replied, 'but they spoil their good looks, you know, by dressing in that absurd Greenaway style'—quite forgetting that she was talking to me.[7]

If Greenaway had made a public comment about the flak the style was receiving, she might very well have pointed out the hypocrisy of the criticism. Though Greenawismes were dubbed too "grown-up," "uncomfortable," and "caricature-like," the same words could easily describe the mainstream fashions of children of the period.

[1.] *Greenaway Book*, p.7
[2.] *Dress*, Mar. 1888, p.595
[3.] *Greenaway Book*, p.8.
[4.] *Child In Fashion*, p.85.
[5.] *La Mode Illustrée*, Sept., 1891
[6.] *Children's Fashions, 1860–1912*, p.2
[7.] *Greenaway Book*, p.24–25.

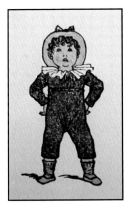

Doll–like children, Greenaway style.

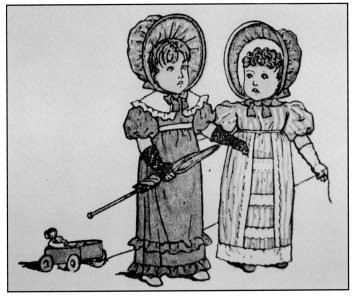

were half–starved, half–frozen, harshly treated, and generally abused—and there were enough true horror stories to back up these fictional accounts. Charlotte Brontë, author of *Jane Eyre* (published in 1847), admitted that her horrifying account of an English boarding school for girls was truthful—and so did many other writers who gave novelized accounts of boarding schools.

"I was called, some weeks ago, to see a young lady who has been for some few years at one of our fashionable boarding–schools not far from Philadelphia," one physician wrote to *Peterson's Magazine* in 1868. "She was a model of beautiful physical health when she was entered at the school, and now returned to her home with an appetite enfeebled and capricious—her digestive functions impaired; her eyes weakened to almost uselessness; her physical strength was all gone; her bright cheek was paled; her spirits depressed—in fact, I was shocked at the change which had come upon her since I saw her last. Her parents were alarmed about her health, and considered her as requiring medical treatment. Upon inquiring into the *regime* of her school, I learned as follows: 'We rise at six, all winter, then read the Bible, and at seven we breakfast, immediately after reading. After breakfast we do up our rooms, and at a quarter before eight we go to the study–rooms, and remain there till nine. At nine we go to the school–room, and remain there until two in the afternoon, except having half an hour recess. At two we dine, leave the table at three, and walk from three to four. From four to seven we study. At seven we have tea. After

tea we study one hour, or read aloud for an hour and a half. We go to bed at ten. We are not allowed to retire earlier. Our courses of study are history, physics, grammar, spelling, arithmetic, algebra, geometry, trigonometry, astronomy, chemistry, Latin, French, German, music, singing, drawing, painting in oil or water colors, and reading aloud from Shakespeare.'...The prescription for the above patient may be easily imagined. Less study; none at all by candlelight; more exercise, and longer rest at night. She is rapidly regaining her former health."

Though the physical requirements of such schools seem harsh, the depth and seriousness of the study was also a matter of deep concern—and the same doctor noted with shock that the school taught neither sewing nor household management.[11] After all, as Victorian writers sometimes stated, future womanly usefulness was endangered by the steady use of the brain.

Yet even while girls' schools were harshly criticized for being too strenuous—and sometimes too studious—many critics also chided them for being frivolous. One caricature from an 1850s issue of *Harper's* pictured the gruesome mistress of a fashionable boarding school, quoting her as saying:

"Our course of studies, did you say, m'm? It is beautifully systematic and regular. At nine in the morning, prayers, with Signor Pregarvi to overlook the kneeling of the young ladies—difficult thing to kneel gracefully with hoops, you know. At ten, one of our French governesses gives her course of *maintien* and deportment. At eleven, singing in Russian and Portuguese, by two eminent exiled Counts. At twelve, Madame Crinoline lectures on the art of dress, with illustrations from nature. We lunch at one, and the Marquis of Jambon instructs the young ladies in habits of refined eating as practiced in aristocratic circles in Europe. At two, visitors—between you and me, young men whom I engage by the month—in order that my young ladies may be perfect in the art of receiving company. At half past three, Signor Bonaventura reads to the boarders for a quarter of an hour a portion of an Italian romance of the most unexceptionable morality. At four, dressing for promenade, under the eye of Madame Crinoline. At five, promenade. At six, dress for dinner, as before. We dine at seven; and the rest of the evening is devoted to light conversation, under the auspices of a poet, a divine, and an ex–foreign ambassador. So you see, our time is pretty well occupied, and we finish our pupils pretty thoroughly.[12]"

But despite the many drawbacks of boarding schools, some sort of "finishing" was generally thought necessary for girls from middle and upper class families. Suggestions ranged from the domestic ("Teach them to be neat, orderly in their habits, and to work...In many cases, mothers will let girls do certain things about housework, while they themselves perform the more difficult tasks...When [their daughters] are married and the whole round of duties falls upon their shoulders, they find it hard to rightly perform those same labors."[13]), to the moral ("You will understand that it really is more important that girls should grow straight than boys."[14]).

Much of the advice given to mothers and teachers in the 19th century about dealing with their daughters and training them to become women focused on how to make them accept their future role in the world.

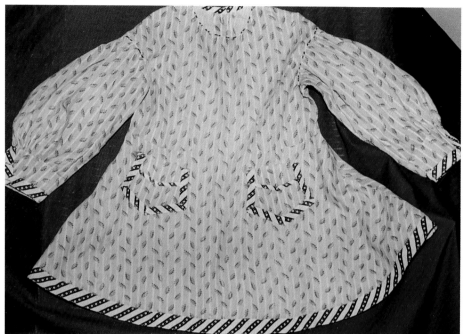
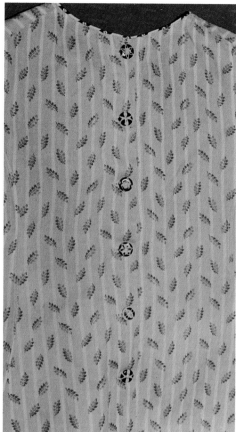

A calico dress, c.1880s—1890s, with six different but matching buttons running down the front. The dress also features contrasting piping at the armhole and neckline, and the same contrasting fabric at the pocket, cuff, and hem. *Courtesy of Pam Coghlan.* $95—$150.

"The other day I heard you and your friend Bessie saying you wished you were boys, because boys have so much freer life than girls, and they grow up into men who can do such great things in the world," the author of *What A Young Girl Ought To Know* wrote.

"The things that men do really do seem very wonderful, but after all they are not greater than the things women do, although they look bigger...Abraham Lincoln, whom we all love as one of the greatest men that ever lived, once said, 'All I am I owe to my mother.' It did not seem that any very great work was being done in that little log cabin when that baby boy was being cared for, but it was beginning his training for the great work he was to accomplish. In the homes all over our land women are busy training boys and girls, bringing them up to be good men and women. Can you think of any greater work than this?...I have read that the battle of Waterloo was lost because of a badly cooked dinner and a consequent indigestion. You see it is possible that the fate of a nation might depend upon a woman's ability to prepare a wholesome meal...Think what we should miss in the way of good times if women were all to go into the world of business away from the world of home...Men are so worried and hurried that they find little time to think about questions of right and wrong, in the world at large; but the wife reads and thinks, and at evenings she says, 'Have you read about the employment of little children in the mills of the South? Really, it is all wrong, and the men who make the laws should be made to feel that the people will not permit such injustice,' and the man begins to think

about this matter...Maybe he does not realize that she is keeping him thinking, but that does not matter, so that he keeps on thinking.[15]"

Other writers and reformers preferred to focus on the physical training of girls. Sometimes this was as simple as making them work hard. *What A Young Girl Ought To Know* also addressed this issue:

"I remember when I was a young woman at boarding school hearing some girls trying to humiliate a new scholar whose hands were red and who looked as if she knew how to work. They were boasting of what they could not do, apparently thinking she would be ashamed of being a working girl.

'Why,' said one of them, 'I never did a stroke of work in my life.'

'Didn't?' said the country girl. 'Don't you know how to wash dishes?'

'Oh, no, indeed!'

'Can't you cook?'

'No.'

'Wash, iron, bake, scrub?'

'No! No!' said the girls, all at once. 'We have servants to do those things.'

'Can't you sew?' asked the country girl.

'Well,' said one of them, 'I made an apron once, but it was so poorly done that my mother had to rip it all out.'

'Well,' said the country girl, 'I would be ashamed to be as helpless as you are—to be like a baby and have some one to wait upon me. You may talk about your fathers being worth money, but I'm worth something myself. I can cook, wash, sew, scrub, bake and iron, and milk and make butter. I am proud of what I can do, and I never would think of boasting about what I can't do.'[16]

But most often, physical training meant—well—gym class. By the late 19th century, gym classes were a common addition to girls schools. Even as early as the 1860s, some boarding schools had special times set aside for tennis or cricket. "In thirty seconds the room is cleared, and we are all upstairs...and putting on knickerbockers and blouses! Yes, *knickerbockers!*" wrote one young woman. "Let no one blush or look shocked, for they are long and ample, and tied modestly at the ankle."[17] Those "shocking" knickerbockers or bloomers were a common sight by the 1890s, when genteel games like cricket were usually replaced with gymnastics and basketball. In Alexander Black's book *Modern Daughters*, where he examines the "New Woman" of the 1890s, an entire chapter is devoted to "The Gym Girl:"

"She herself wore a dark serge gym suit, that fascinating hybrid of skirt and bloomer, which unites the charm of drapery with the effect of the girded uniform. Sitting there thus well–dressed, lithe, poised, sufficient, with light in her eyes and blood in her lips, she presented a pleasing spectacle. Something in her association with all the paraphernalia of the vaulted gymnasium struck me as symbolizing the situation of her sex in the modern world...

'I suppose you think all this is very absurd,' said the Gym Girl, tapping the floor with her slipper. 'Sometimes I myself think it is. But I like it; I like it well enough not to care what anyone thinks, and besides, I am supported by the moments when I think it isn't a bit absurd...What idea does the gym represent?' she asked in a tone of challenge.

[I answered] 'In the city it is very different for all of us, but especially for you women. The clothes you usually wear here presuppose that you will suspend, while wearing them, the use or development of most of your muscles. Some of the time you will wear a bicycle skirt and ride a wheel. But the bicycle uses but one set of muscles. Your walking and dancing, with some tennis and

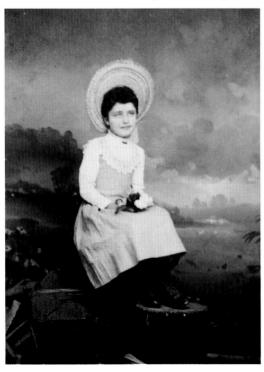

A picturesque photo of a girl from the 1880s adorned with lace, a straw bonnet, high button boots, and flowers.

an occasional run out to the links for gold, all leave the symmetrical development incomplete in some way...The gymnasium ought to fill in the chinks...Then it makes you like it.'

'It does make me like it, because it makes me like myself. The gymnasium makes me feel good—*good*, do you understand, not merely *well*.'[18]"

It was not just girls that were forced into the drudgery of learning household management and other "life skills," however. Boys were often trained to be protective toward their sisters and mothers, to spend money wisely, and even to do basic sewing. "We must see that boys are early taught to sew," Elizabeth Stanton, one of the early feminists, argued. She felt that not only should boys learn the traditional skill of clothes–mending, but that they should be trained to completely create and sew all their own clothes. "I see no reason why boys should be left to roam the streets day and night, wholly unemployed, a nuisance to everybody and a curse to themselves, while their sisters are over–taxed at home to make and mend their brothers' clothes. It will be a glorious day for the emancipation of those of our sex who have long been slaves to the needle, when men and boys make their own clothes..."[19]

While boys were expected to take on—even if only in a cursory way—manly attributes at the early age of breeching, girls waited to adopt adult attributes until the difficult years of puberty. Many American girls (at least those not belonging to the fashionable class) were allowed to roam rather freely, like boys, until their bodies began to show the first signs of womanliness. Lucy Larcom, writing of her New England girlhood, noted that this seemed a natural American right. "We did not think those English children [from books] had so good a time as we did; they had to be so prim and methodical. It seemed to us that the little folks across the water never were allowed to romp and run wild...[we had] a vague idea that this freedom of ours was the natural inheritance of republican children only."[20]

The autobiographies of 19th century American girls make it seem that half the population of little girls of the period were what would be deemed Tom Boys. "I often climbed trees and tore my clothes," wrote one woman of her childhood. Una Hunt, writing of the 1870s–80s, also bragged that she climbed "every tree and shed in the neighborhood. I was often badly hurt, but after each fall, vinegar and brown papers had been applied, [and my mother's] only comment was 'You must learn to climb better,' and I did."[21] In fact, some Victorian writers even admitted that "little tykes often turn out smart women."[22]

Not all little girls were allowed such freedom, however. Girls from wealthy families were frequently trained from an early age to be little ladies, and a girl of any class might make an early entrance into womanhood if her mother died and she was left in charge of the household. Too, not everyone thought it a good idea to encourage rambunctious behavior in girls. "That bold, enterprising spirit, which is so much admired in boys, should not, when it happens to discover itself in the other sex, be encouraged," one writer cautioned in 1777. "Girls should be taught to give up their opinions betimes...It is of the greatest importance to their future happiness, that they should acquire a submissive tempter, and a forbearing spirit; for it is a lesson the world will not fail to make them frequently practice, when they come abroad into it, and they will not practice it the worse for having learnt it the sooner."[23]

The age when girls of all ranks were expected to change into womanhood varied, but it began at thirteen, and was expected to have been achieved by fifteen—and certainly no later than sixteen. Like boys, this change into adulthood had more to do with the size and shape of the body than it did with age. "No girl went through a harder experience than I, when my free, out–of–door life had to cease, and the long skirts and blubbed–up hair spiked with hairpins had to be endured," wrote Francis Willard (founder of the Women's Christian Temperance Union) of this transition. "The half of that down–heartedness has never been told and never can be. I always believed that if I had been left alone and allowed as a woman what I had as a girl, a free life in this country, where a human being might grow, body and soul, as a tree grows, I would have been ten times more of a person in every way." To stress this point, Willard even went so far as to excerpt what she said was a page from her girlhood diary: "This is my birthday and the date of my martyrdom. Mother insists that at least I must have my hair 'done up woman–fashion.' My 'back' hair is twisted up like a corkscrew. I carry eighteen hairpins; my head aches miserably; my feet are entangled in the skirt of my hateful new gown. I can never jump over a fence again, so long as I live."[24] Willard was not the only woman to complain so bitterly. "The transition from childhood to girlhood, when a girl had an almost unlimited freedom of out–of–door life, is practically the toning down of a mild sort of barbariansim," Lucy Larcom wrote. "I clung to the child's inalienable privilege of running half wild; and when I found that I really was growing up, I felt quite rebellious."[25]

*Clothes For The Prairie*

"While traveling, mother was particular about Louvina and me wearing sunbonnets and long mitts in order to protect our complexions, hair and hands," wrote Adrietta Hixon, speaking of her childhood journey West in the 1850s. "Much of the time I should like to have gone without that long bonnet poking out over my face, but mother pointed out to me some girls who did not wear bonnets and as I did not wish to look as they did, I stuck to my bonnet finally growing used to it."[1] Indeed, the experience of traveling to and settling in the West in the 19th century required a whole new outlook on clothing.

Most often, this new outlook simply meant taking fashionable styles and making them out of durable, practical cottons and wools rather than silks or velvets. But it also meant simplification: Hoopskirts were taboo, a mass of ruffles and furbelows were definitely discouraged, and clothing would have to be mended and re–mended many times before it was discarded. "In jumping off the horse alone today, I caught my dress in the horn of the saddle and tore almost half of the skirt off," another young immigrant woman wrote. "I have had no dress on since the day we came to Westport but my...muslin delaine [a wool/cotton blend]. I mean to stick to it as long as I can. It is very dirty and has been torn nearly if not quite twenty times."[2] But despite the fact that so–called "prairie" clothing was often worn until it wore out, a surprising amount of it still exists today.

[1] *Women's Diaries*, p.84
[2] ibid., p.101

For boys, the change into young adulthood—though it often came earlier—was accepted with more pride because it offered the boy more freedom. But for girls, young adulthood meant less freedom—and after thirteen or more years of tasting it. Nonetheless, while the majority of autobiographies, diaries, and letters reveal that girls despised this change into adulthood, some girls felt the opposite. "I hated being a child," silent film star Gloria Swanson wrote. "In those days there was no such thing as a teenager in between. I couldn't wait to wear long skirts and put my hair up on top of my head and wear a wedding ring and be Mrs. Somebody with twelve children—six on each side of the dining–room table."[26]

Generally in the 19th century, from the ages of four to nine girls' skirts were worn so that they reached the top of their high–button boots; at ten years, the skirt was about half-way between the knees and the tops of their shoes. And by the age of sixteen to eighteen, a girl's skirts dropped to the floor, making her fit for courting. "If the health of a girl is sound, the marriageable age should be from twenty to twenty–five or six years," *Demorest's Monthly Magazine* advised in 1887. "If they have been weakened by overstudy or too much physical labor, the forces should have full time to recover their equilibrium before entering upon this ordeal; for the happiness of families is best secured by the sound health of parents."[27]

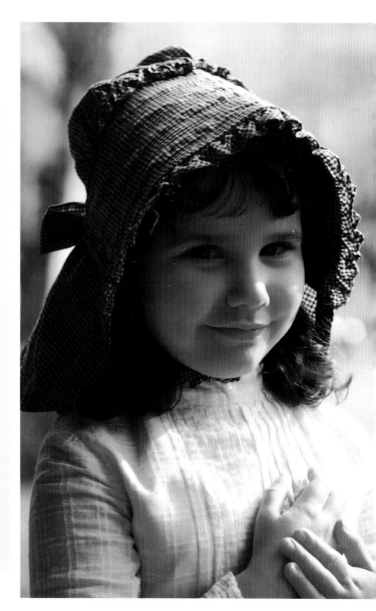

## Endnotes:

1. *The Delineator*, Oct. 1905
2. *Fabulous Century*, p.8–9
3. *Children's Costume in America*, p.194
4. *Fabulous Century*, p.124
5. *Everyday Life*, p.129
6. James McCabe *Lights And Shadows of New York Life*, 1872, p. 833–834
7. *Century of Childhood*, p.74
8. *The Delinator*, Oct.1905, p.577
9. *De Vicilitate morum puerilium* ("Manners for Children") by Erasmus, 1530; *History of Private Life*, p.184
10. *The Delineator*, Oct.1905, p. 577
11. *Peterson's Magazine*, June 1868, p.466
12. *Harper's Weekly*, 1857
13. *The Household*, Feb.1882, p.50
14. *What A Young Girl....*, p.124
15. ibid., p.171–77
16. ibid., p.131–32
17. *History of Children's Costume*, p.117–118
18. *Modern Daughters*, p.43–46
19. *Bloomer Girls*, p.43–44
20. *A New England Girlhood*, p.104
21. *Reminiscences of Newcastle, Iowa*, p.180; *Una May*, p. 47
22. *Jack & Jill*, p.220
23. *Century of Childhood*, p.118
24. *American Woman*, p.69
25. *New England Girlhood*, p. 166–67
26. *Swanson*, p.14
27. *Demorest's Monthly Magazine*, June 1887, p.499

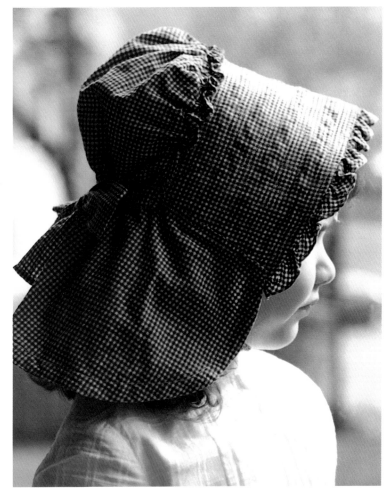

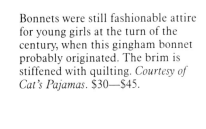

Bonnets were still fashionable attire for young girls at the turn of the century, when this gingham bonnet probably originated. The brim is stiffened with quilting. *Courtesy of Cat's Pajamas*. $30—$45.

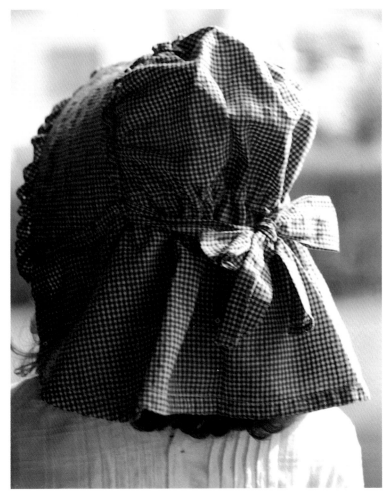

*Lessons For Little Gentlemen And Ladies*

"A lady in society must, if she would not grow utterly weary in company, know how to dance," *The Ladies Book of Etiquette* advised in the mid–19th century. "There is nothing immoral or wrong in dancing; it is the tendency of youth to dance—it is the first effort of a child—the first natural recreation."[1] Indeed, any parent who hoped his or her child would grow into a lady or gentleman suited for society made certain their child received dancing lessons. No doubt like many well–to–do parents, in letters to his son Lord Chesterfield asked: "Do you mind your dancing while your dancing master is with you?"[2] Dancing was such an important social activity, in fact, that learning to dance could not be left to chance; private lessons given by male instructors were most popular among the wealthy, but even middle–class boarding schools offered dancing lessons.

"In the present day, you must understand how to move gracefully through quadrilles, to dance polka, Schottische, Varsovienne, and waltz. To these you may add [a] great variety of dances, each season probably, bringing a new one," the editors of *The Ladies Book Of Etiquette* wrote. Still, learning to dance properly was not as easy as might first be thought; there were numerous rules for dancing like a gentleman or lady. Even the waltz—one of the most basic of all dances—had to be done in such a way that no one could suspect the dancers' morality was dubious. "The position is a most important point," *The Ladies Book of Etiquette* pointed out. "You may so lean upon your partner's arm, and so carry your figure, that the prudish can find but little fault, but you can also make the dance a most immodest one..."[3] After all, in the 18th and 19th centuries, to learn to dance properly was the first step toward a successful social life.

[1] *Ladies' Book of Etiquette,* p.198
[2] *Martine's,* p.92
[3] *Ladies' Book of Etiquette,* p.199–204

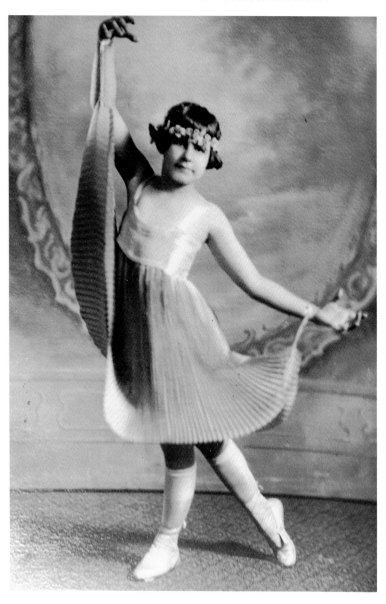

The tradition of dancing school extended somewhat into the 1920s—though by then, the focus was definitely more on girls than on boys. This girl from the 20s posed for the photographer in her ballet costume.

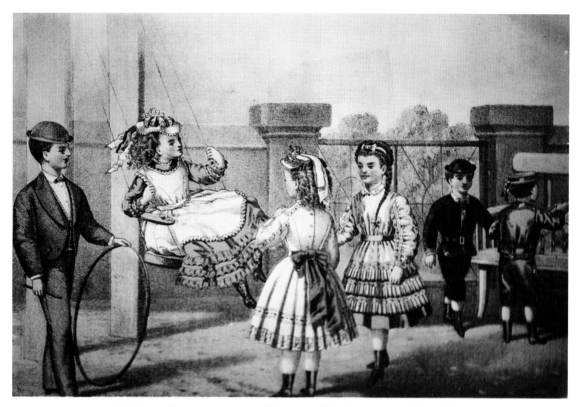

Children's fashions from an 1871 issue of *The Metropolitan*. $50—$75.

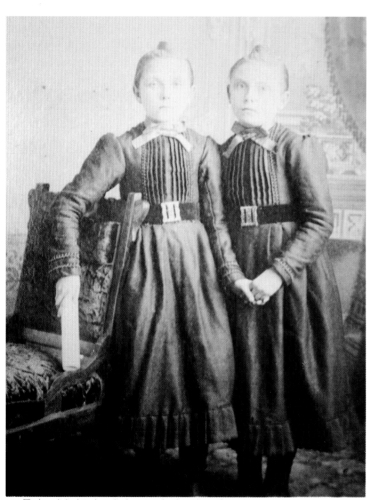

Twin girls in simple but typical attire of the early 1870s.

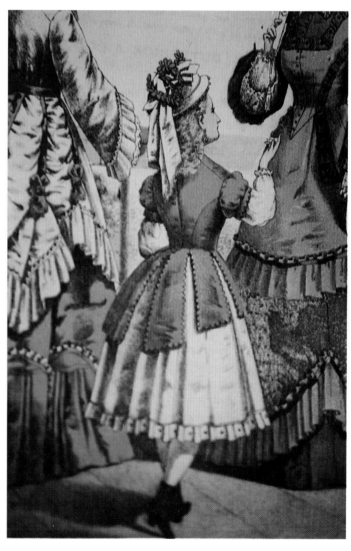

An 1871 fashion plate showing a girl wearing a white mohair skirt
worn with a pink silk over–dress that fastens with tiny buttons down
the back. $45—$65.

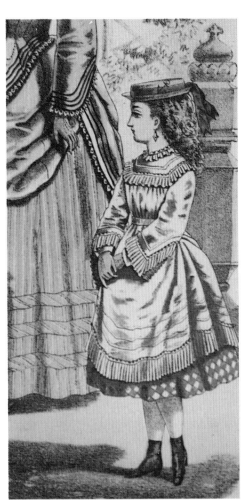

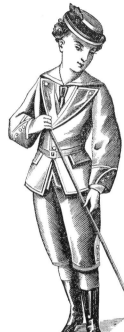

An 1871 fashion plate featuring a girl's typical attire. $45—$65.

*Godey's Lady's Book* pictured this boy's suit in the 1870s.

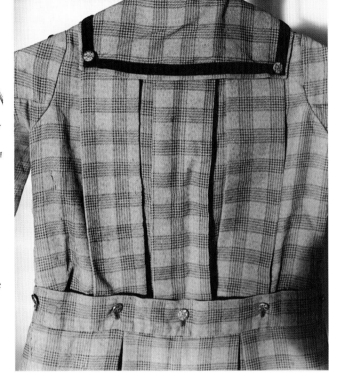

A c. 1870–1880 boy's wool plaid dress. Like most boy's dresses of the period, although it appears to be two–piece, with the skirt buttoning onto a dropped waist, it is actually one piece. All the buttons, except those running down the front of the bodice, are purely decorative. The dress is trimmed with black silk velvet and lace. *Courtesy of Vintage Silhouettes.* $100—$150.

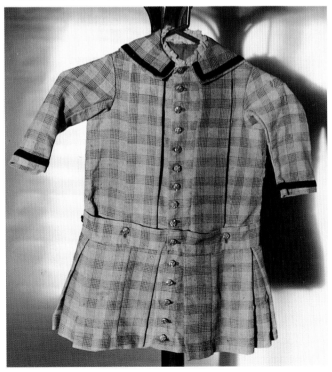

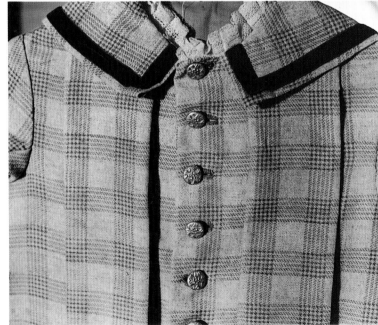

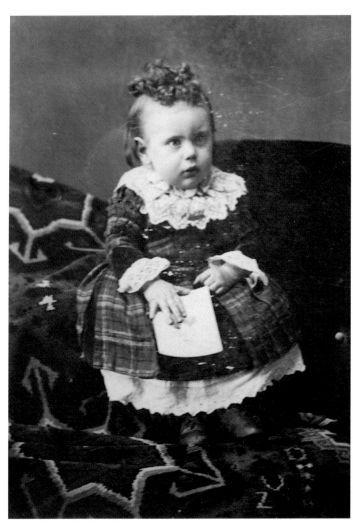

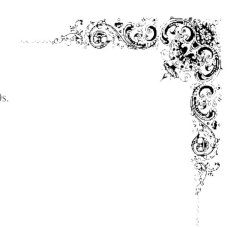

A little boy from the 1870s.

Typical toddler attire of the early 1870s.

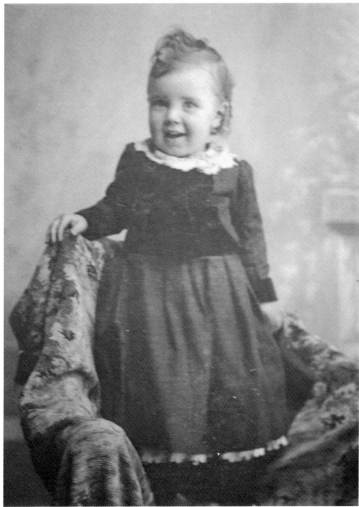

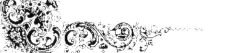

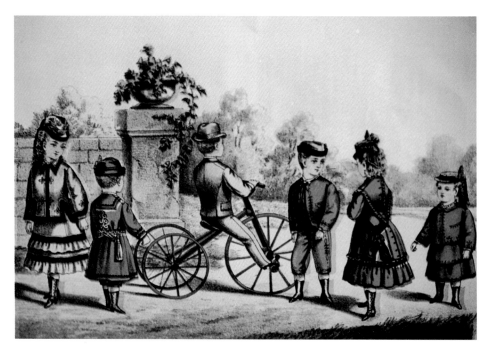

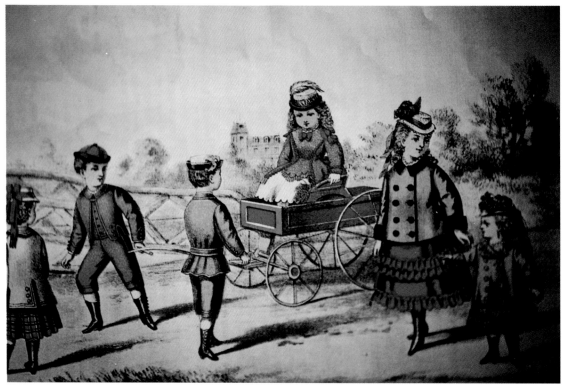

Children's fashions from 1873. Each of these patterns could be purchased through Butterick at 10¢ to 30¢ a piece. $50—$75.

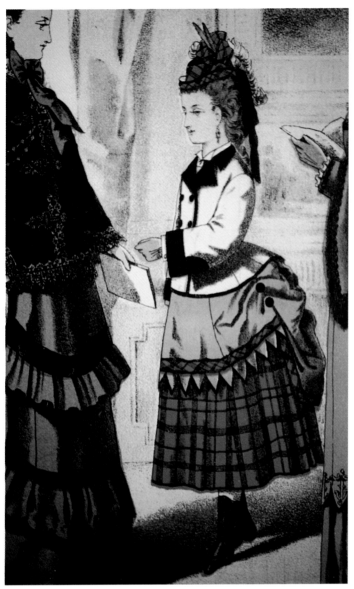

A baby's dress from the early 1870s.

Butterick patterns' *Metropolitan* magazine featured this girl's dress in 1873, describing it as a "pretty suit of three kinds of materials." The skirt is of plaid serge, while the over–skirt is of wool and is looped up creating a bustle effect by the aid of buttons. The bodice is also wool and is trimmed with velvet. $45—$60.

A c.1878–1885 baby's dress of cotton with an eyelet collar. An inset of gathering in the back gives the dress a slight bustle effect; the front of the dress is plain. *Courtesy of Vintage Silhouettes.* $45—$65.

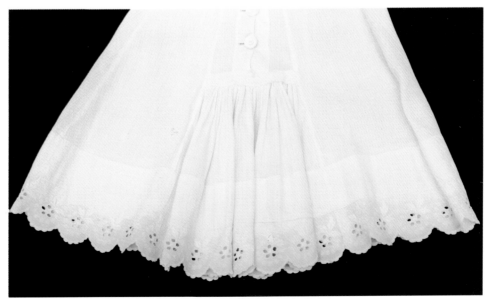

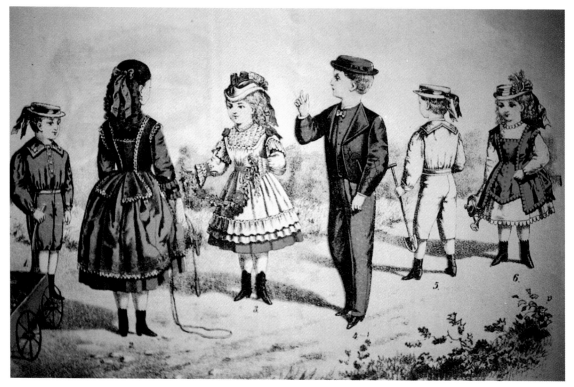

A children's fashion plate from 1871. Notice that while all the girls are dressed similarly, only the eldest boy wears a scaled down man–style suit. $50—$75.

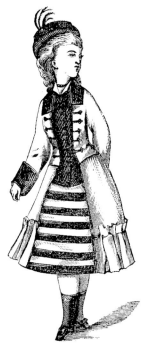

A dress for a twelve year old girl, from an 1870s fashion plate. $45—$65.

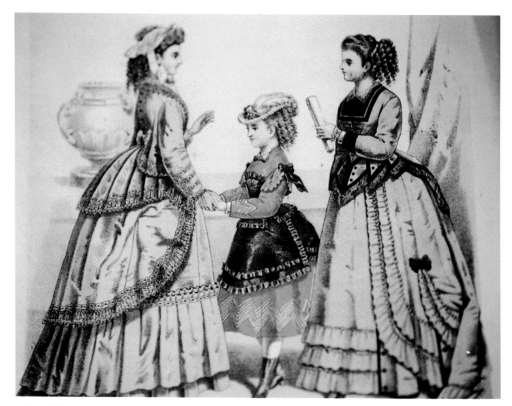

This 1871 fashion plate shows just how similar girls' and womens' fashions were during this period. Unlike her mother, however, the girl shown here wears considerably more comfortable, shorter skirts. Boys, on the other hand, only dressed as miniature men after they reached a particular age. $50—$75.

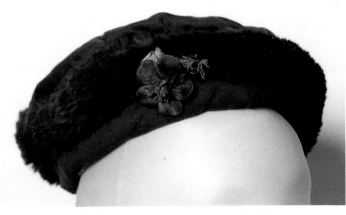

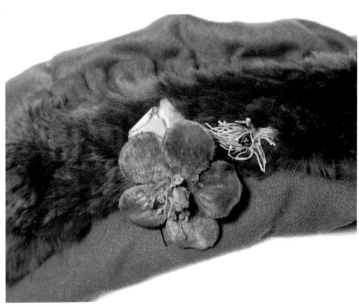

A c.1878 girl's hat of wool trimmed with fur and a fabric pansy. *Courtesy of Antique Apparel.* $45—$85.

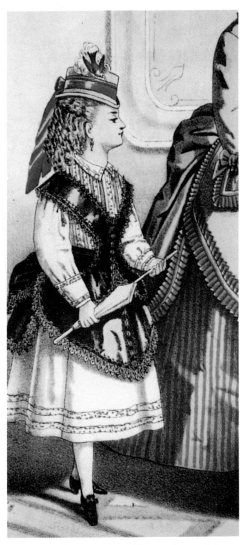

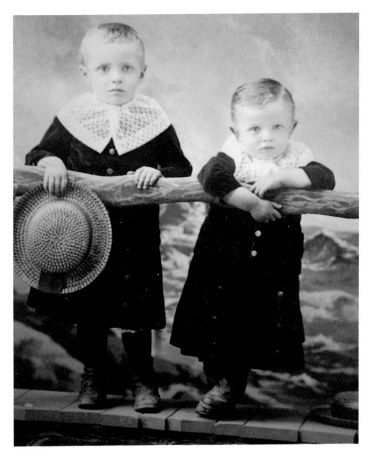

Boys from the 1870s, wearing velvet dresses trimmed with lace.

An 1872 fashion plate, illustrating a girl's silk dress consisting of three pieces: Skirt, blouse, and over–dress. The pattern could be purchased through Butterick for 45¢. $45—$65.

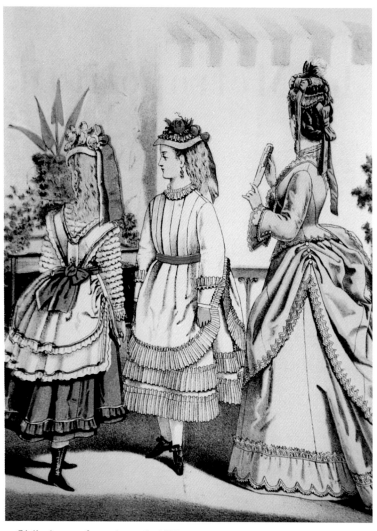

Girl's dresses from the early 1870s.

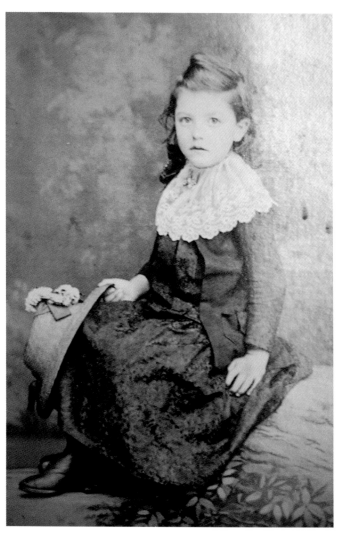

A fashionable girl of the 1880s wearing a silk dress trimmed with a wide lace collar, a slight bustle, and a straw hat.

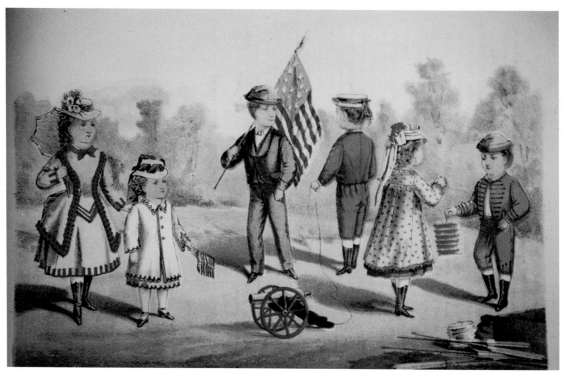

An 1872 children's fashion plate. $50—$75.

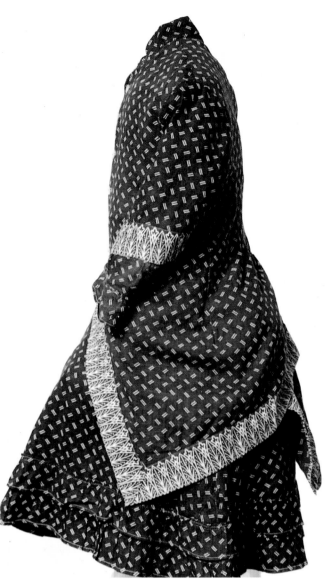

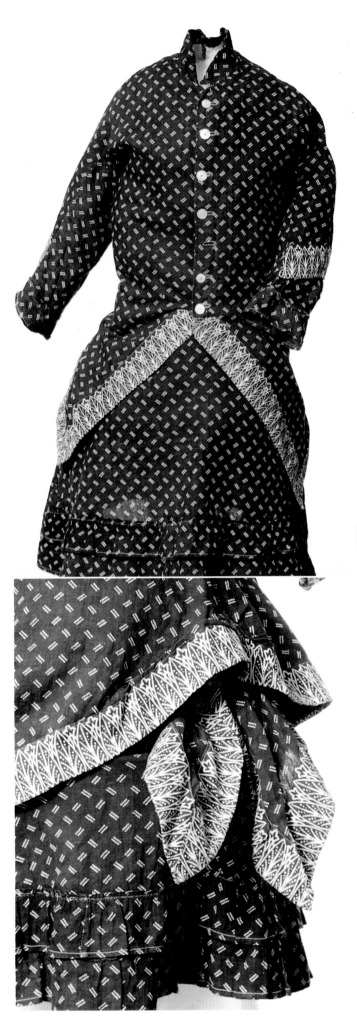

A c.1880s two-piece calico dress with border trim on the hem of the bodice and appliqué border trims on the sleeves. A separate piece of material is sewn onto the bodice at center back, which helps give the bustle effect. *Courtesy of Pam Coghlan.* $195—$300.

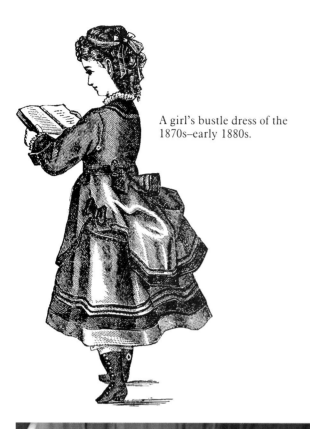

A girl's bustle dress of the 1870s–early 1880s.

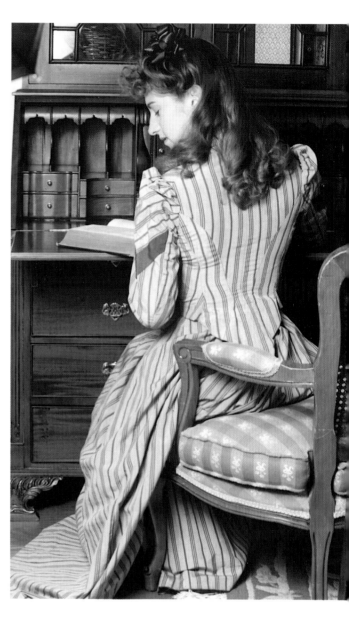

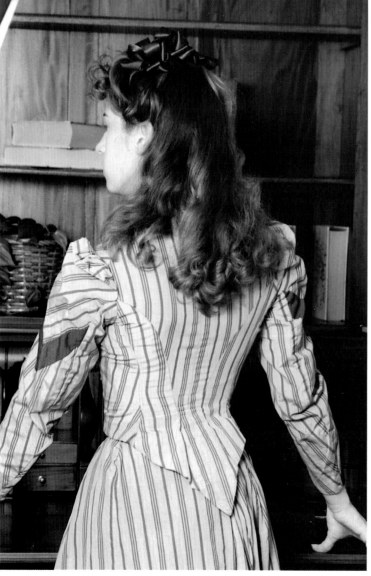

A typical c.1889–1891 misses' two–piece dress. The bodice is snug–fitting with hooks and eyes down the front; the heavy skirt is fully gathered. *Courtesy of Vintage Silhouettes.* $150—$250.

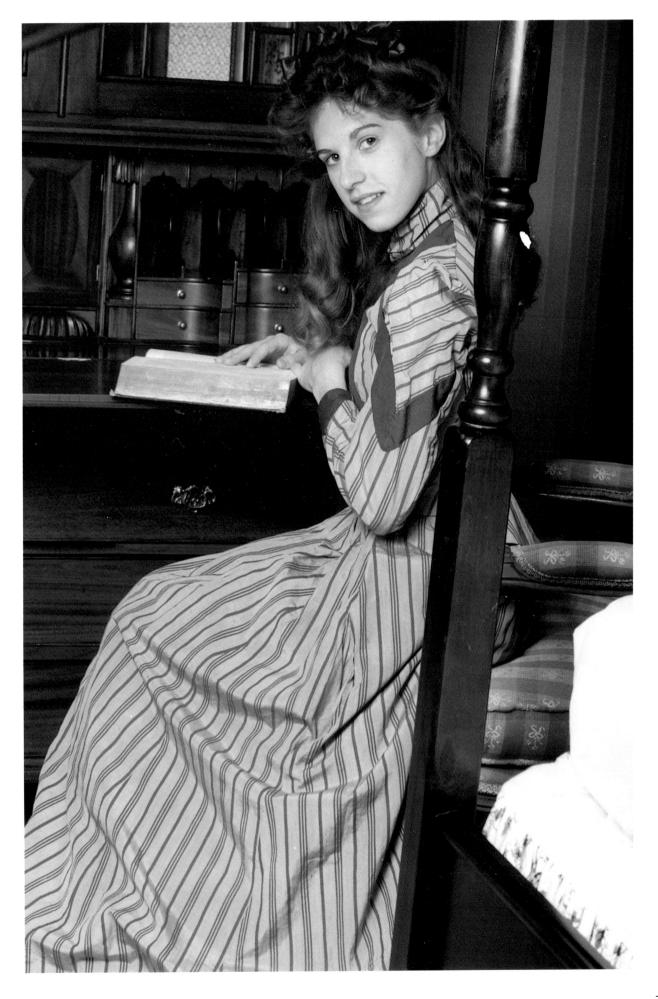

Boys' dresses from 1886.

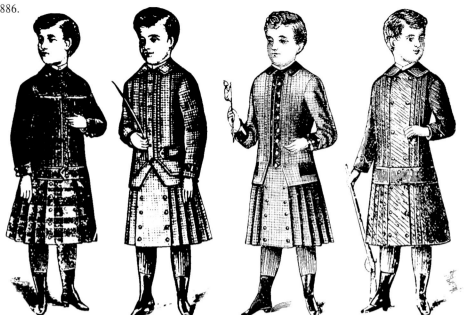

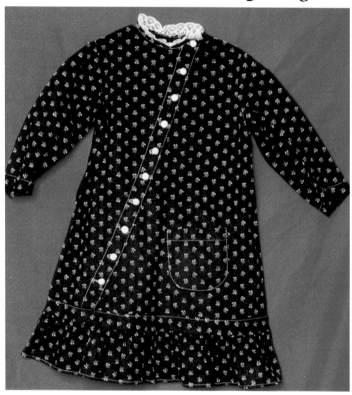

The simplicity of trimmings and asymmetrical front button closure of this calico dress indicates that it was designed for a boy. The dress comes with a handwritten note: "This is a dress Mother was making for Wade when he died—about 1 1/2 years old in Nov. 1885." *Courtesy of Pam Coghlan.* With note $175—$250; without note $95—$125.

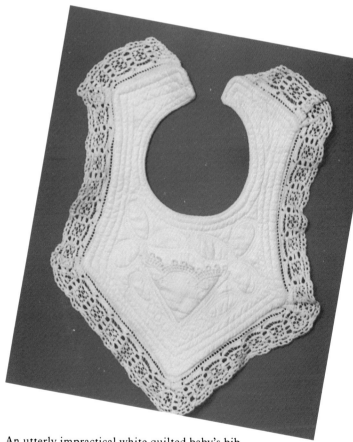

An utterly impractical white quilted baby's bib c.1887–1915. It is trimmed with lace, and at center front features a tiny pocket. It measures approximately 10 inches long by 7.5 inches wide. *Courtesy of Pam Coghlan.* $25—$65.

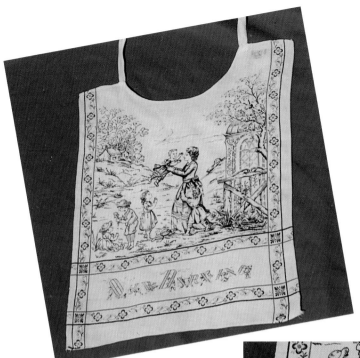

Decorative baby bibs were popular throughout the 19th century. This printed bib dates to the last half of the 19th century, and measures approximately 11 inches wide by 13.5 inches long. *Courtesy of Pam Coghlan.* $100—$185.

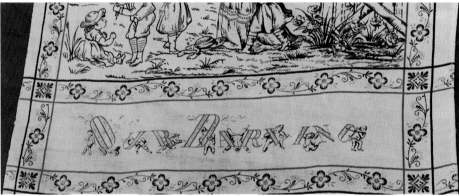

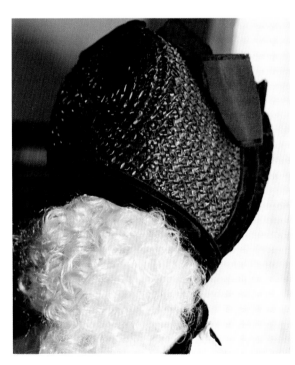

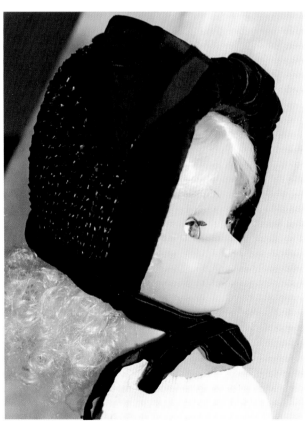

A c.1880s girl's straw bonnet with black velvet trim and a blue ribbon bow on top. *Courtesy of Vintage Silhouettes.* $100—$140.

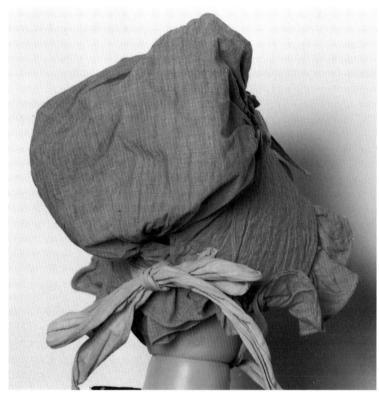

A c.1880–1905 chambray bonnet whose only embellishments are quilting and a front and center bow. *Courtesy of Pam Coghlan.* $55—$75.

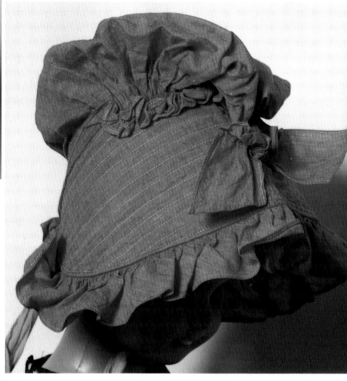

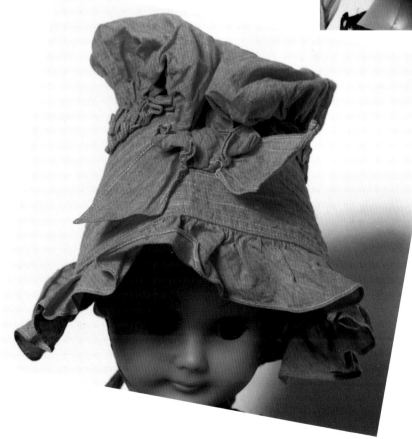

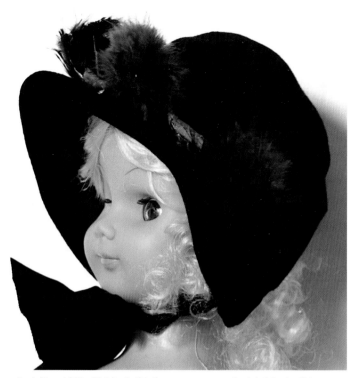

A girl's c.1880–90 black felt bonnet accented with black ribbon ties and green feathers. *Courtesy of Mother & Daughter Vintage.* $50—$70.

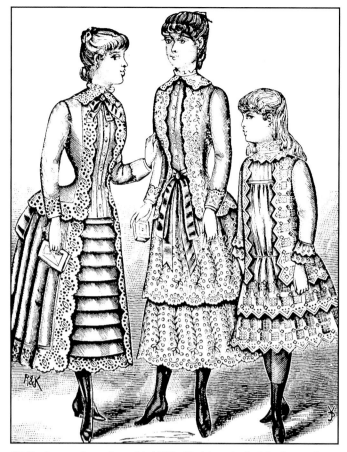

Girl's dresses from the mid–1880s. Fashioned of white lawn, they could be purchased ready–made for $3.95—$13.50 each.

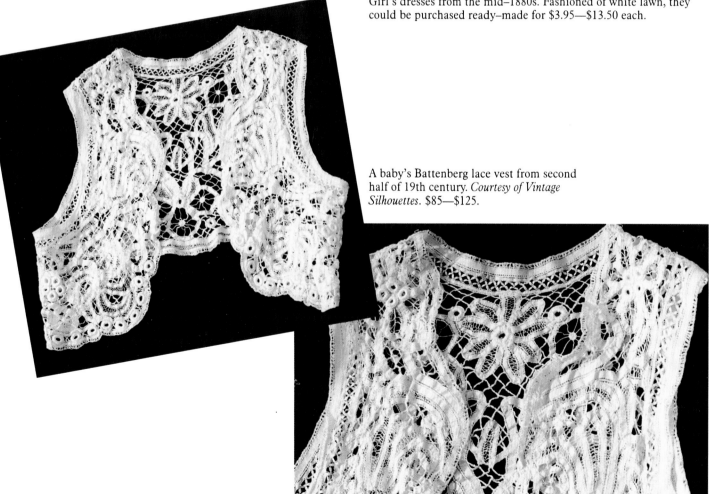

A baby's Battenberg lace vest from second half of 19th century. *Courtesy of Vintage Silhouettes.* $85—$125.

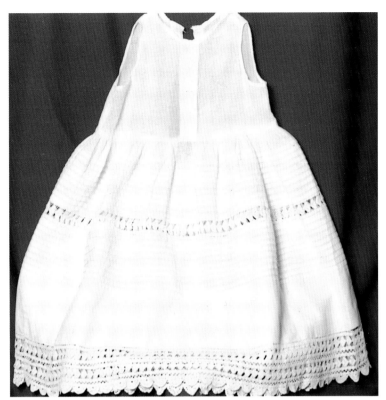

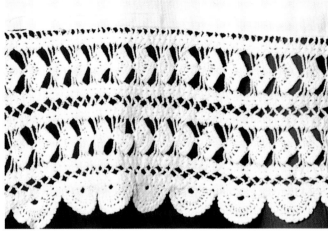

A c.late 1880s–1890s baby's slip with a typically plain, sleeveless bodice and a gathered skirt featuring many pintucks and crochet insertion trim. There are no buttons, hooks and eyes, or snaps for fastening the slip; it would have originally been closed with pins. *Courtesy of The Very Little Theatre.* $10—$25.

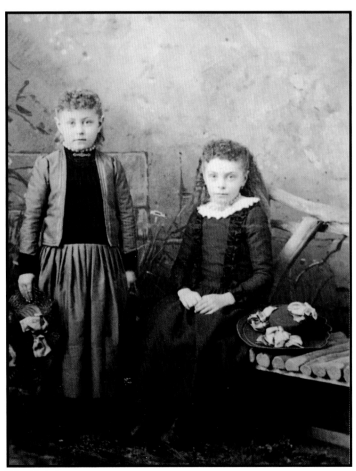

Sisters dressed in mid–1880s attire. The look is harsh, but fashionable, and the dresses fit better than most period photos of the era indicate was typical.

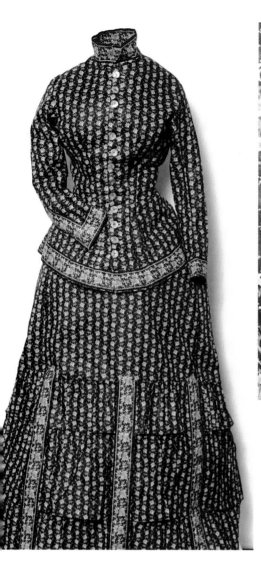

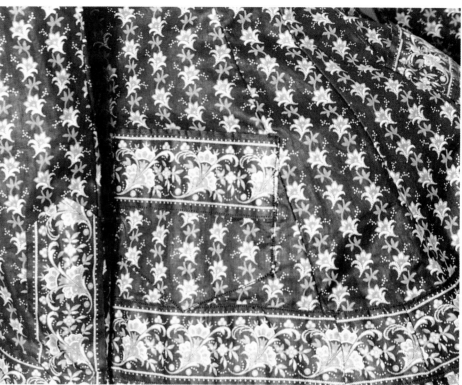

A bold two–piece calico dress, c.1880s. This is a beautifully made garment, which still has sizing in the fabric, indicating that it was never washed—and probably never worn. The mandarin collar leads to 14 abalone buttons down the front, and extra fullness is allowed for the bustle effect in back. The separate skirt is gathered with most of the fullness at back; there is a pocket hidden in the seams of the skirt. This garment also shows wonderful use of border prints: on the collar, pocket, hem of bodice, sleeve, and skirt waistband. In addition, there is an unusual hem trimming; three ruffles are featured on the skirt, but are tacked down with bands of the border print. *Courtesy of Pam Coghlan.* $250—$400.

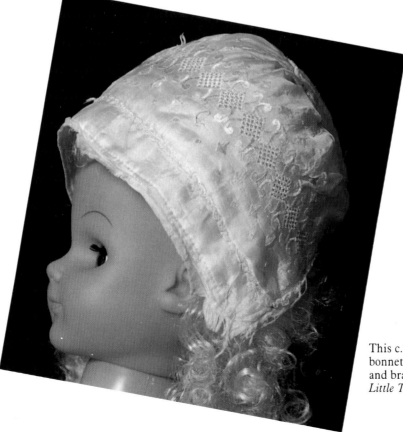

This c.late 1880s–1890s silk baby bonnet features extensive embroidery and braid trim. *Courtesy of The Very Little Theatre.* $10—$25.

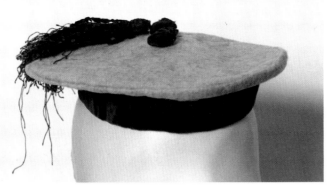

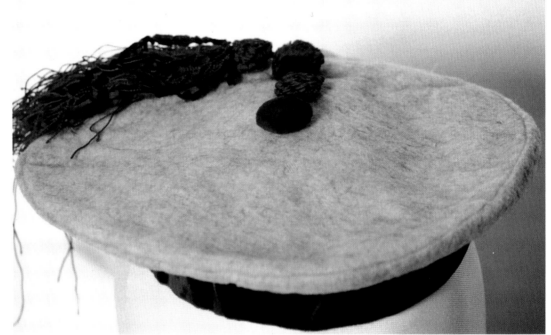

A c.1880s–1890s hat of brown felt with a tiny bill, a band of maroon velvet, and a maroon tassel topping it off. It was probably worn by a girl. *Courtesy of Antique Apparel.* $20—$50.

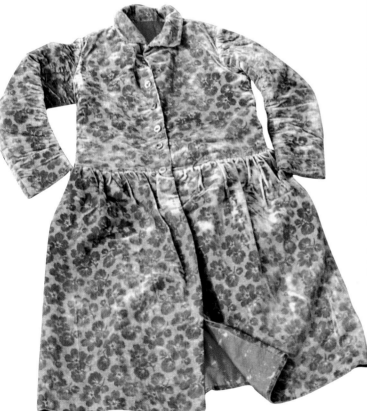

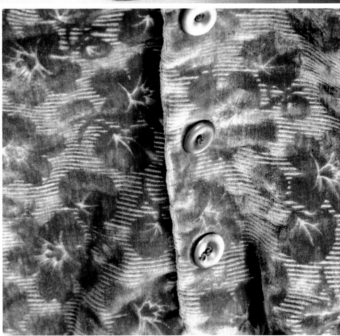

An unusual girl's coat, c.1880s–90s. This coat appears to have originally been a shorter jacket, with the skirt of the coat sewn on later—although the entire garment on outside is the same silk velvet fabric. The bodice buttons up the front and is lined with quilted red satin. The waistline seam features a peplum on the inside where the skirt of the coat is sewn on. The skirt, which is open in front, is lined in red silk/wool blend. *Courtesy of Antique Apparel.* $50—$75.

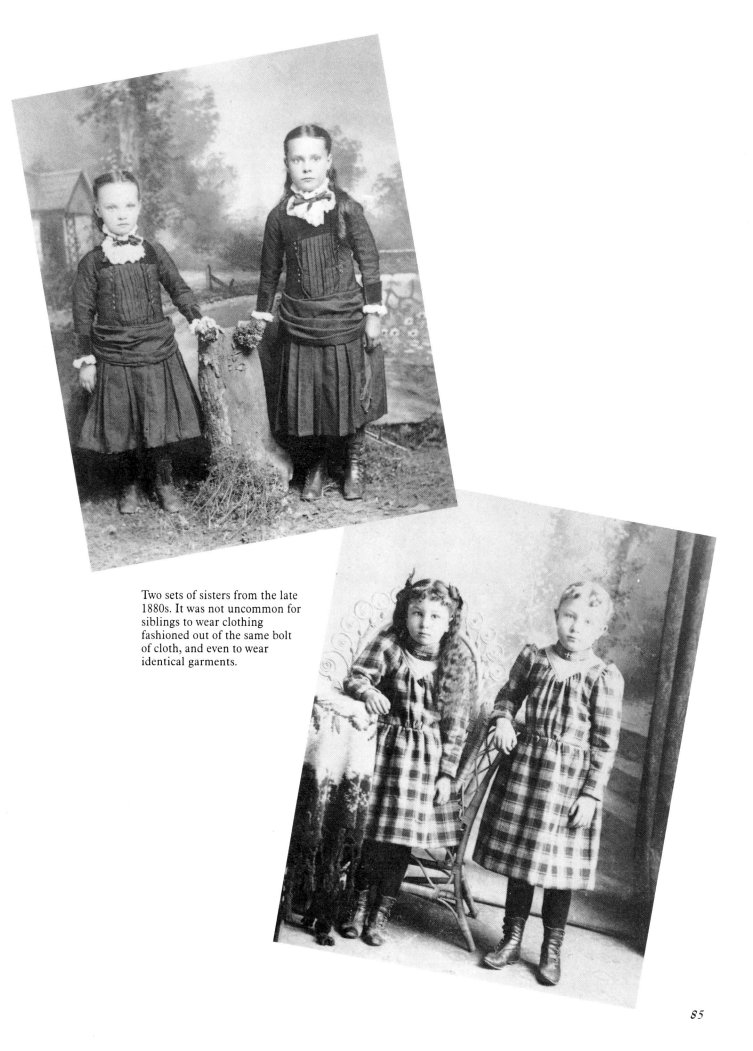

Two sets of sisters from the late 1880s. It was not uncommon for siblings to wear clothing fashioned out of the same bolt of cloth, and even to wear identical garments.

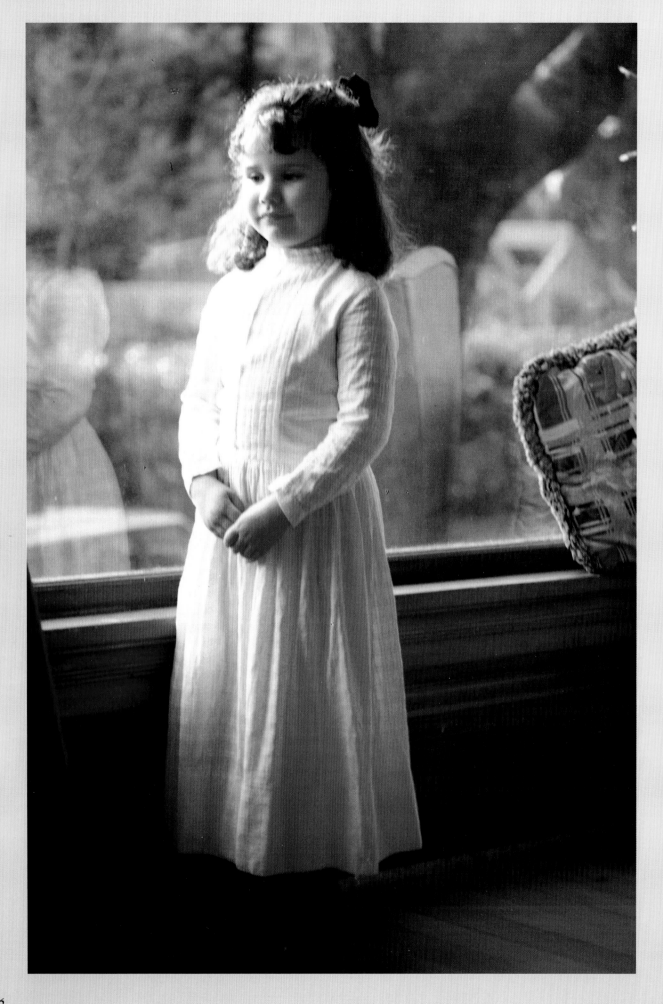

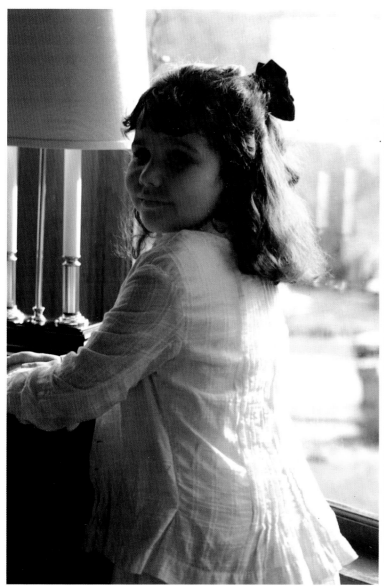

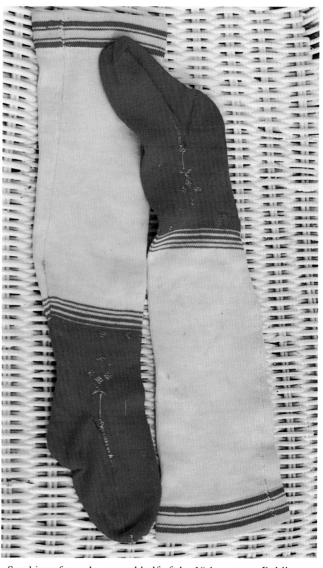

Stockings from the second half of the 19th century. Boldly garnished with red stripes, and with red feet trimmed with white embroidery, they are typical of the 1860s–1880s. *Courtesy of Antique Apparel.* $95—$140.

This girl's dress from the turn of the century features a tucked front, an attached gathered skirt, and buttons running up the back. The separate jacket is very similar to the dress bodice, with tucks all across the front. *Courtesy of Vintage Silhouettes.* $25—$55.

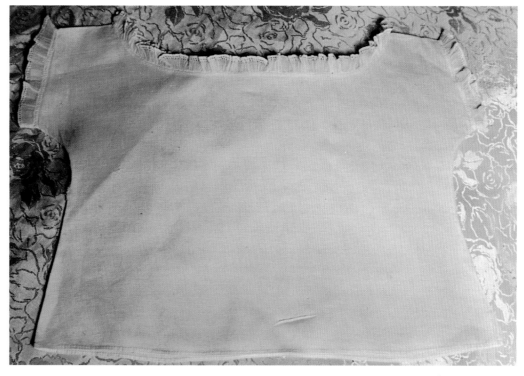

An infant's shirt, c.1880s–1890s. Its only trimming are the slight ruffles along the neckline and sleeves. *Courtesy of Antique Apparel.* $10—$35.

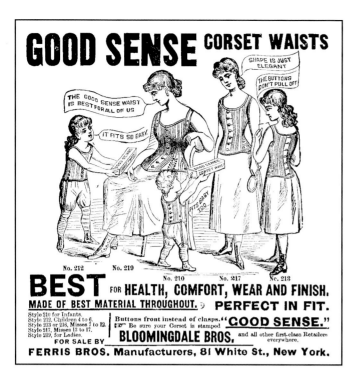

An 1880s ad for corsets for the ages: for infants, young children, young miss', and women.

This manufacturer specialized in corsets for children, emphasizing the comfort and practicality of their styles. This full page ad appeared in an 1888 issue of *Dress*.

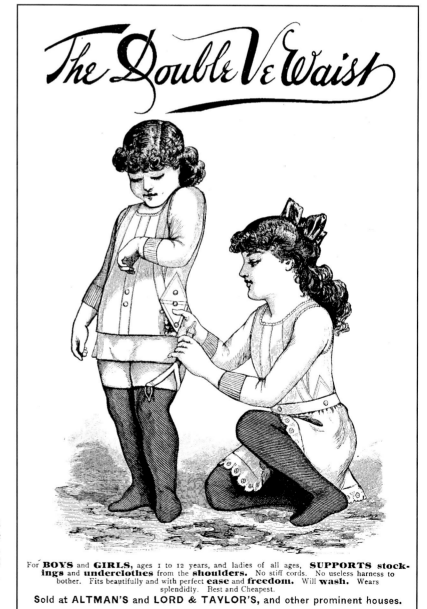

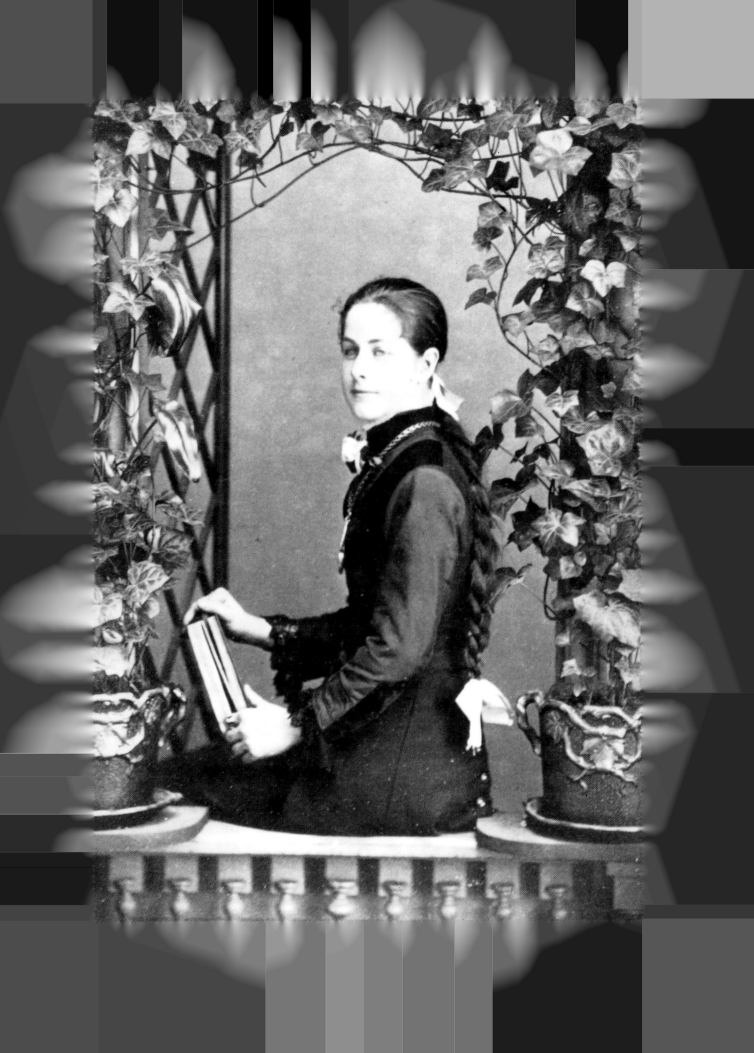

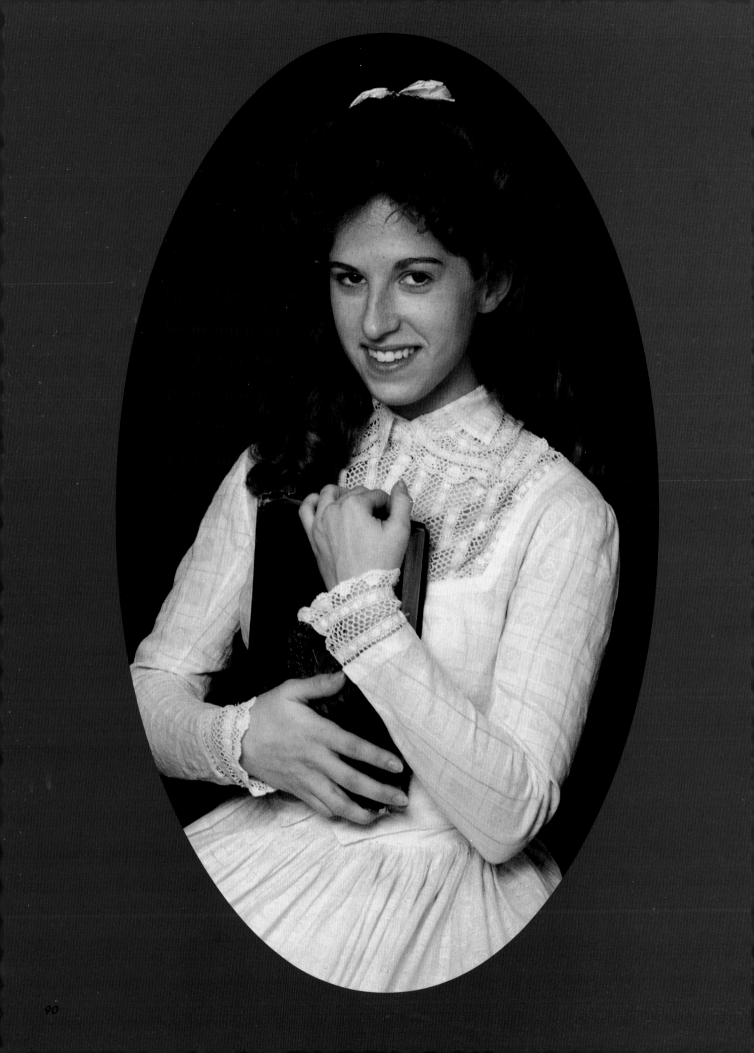

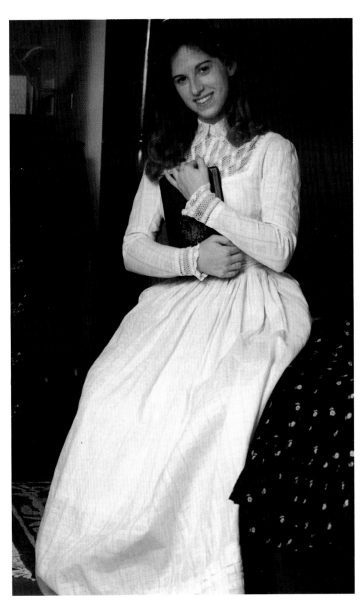

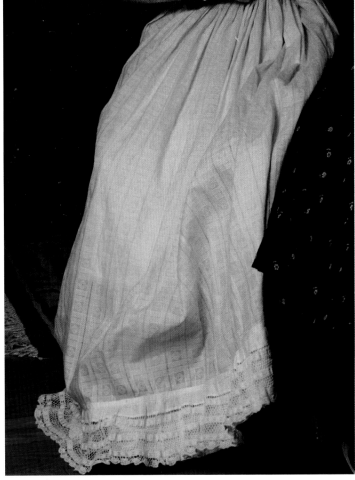

This white cotton dress, c.1888–1890, is actually two–piece. The skirt is very full and gauged tightly into the waistband. The bodice buttons up the front, and features a yolk of faggoting. The sleeve ends and the hem of the skirt are both trimmed with faggoting and ruffles. *Courtesy of Vintage Silhouettes.* $200—$360.

# In The Guise of Play

"The tiniest of school girls [are] miniature women with ruffles and large sleeves, making each little tot nearly as broad as she is long," *Ladies Home Journal* commented in the 1890s.[1] As it had been in the early 1800s, little girls were dressing as near miniatures of their mothers. The huge sleeves, gored skirts—and even the high collars—of fashionable women's attire could also be glimpsed in youthful attire. Fortunately, however, a more comfortable and practical style prevailed for many young girls, also: The smock dress. "For little girls from about four to nine the most universally approved styles are those having a yoke—whether square or round—into which the material is gathered. No trimming is used at the hem, but three small tucks are useful for letting down at some future date," one source advised in 1892.[2] Some smock dresses were sleeved, but many were sleeveless and meant to be worn with a blouse—usually a properly starched white blouse. Smock dresses were, however, nothing new; they had been worn by country folks for decades. But when Walter Crane, a children's book illustrator, drew smock dresses for an English magazine, followed by illustrations in the increasingly–popular American reform journals, the smock burst into the world of fashionable attire. Still, after age nine or so, girls' waists were usually marked with a waistband or sash.

"What I, on behalf off my fifty–years ago self may envy the little girls of today is the fewness and simplicity of their garments," wrote Eleanor Acland in her autobiography. "We, too, put on first of all a vest [for warmth]. Then a chemise, a garment, whose use was never apparent to us, but we were given to understand that it wouldn't be at all 'nice' to go without it. It was made of calico and reached the knees. Next 'stays,' a strip of wadded pique whose use was unmistakable. In addition to the five buttons that fastened our stays up the back, they had a number of other buttons at various levels and intervals round the waist. Two of these held up the elastic 'spenders' of our stockings; the five buttonholes of our drawers belonged to the other three, and yet two more were buttoned into two holes in the band of our flannel petticoat. Over that came a white petticoat made with a bodice. The edges of all the white garments were decorated with rather scratchy cambric trimming..."[3] Other necessities to the turn of the century girl's dress included gloves. These, though it is difficult for us to imagine today, were worn even by small children whenever they were out of doors in anything other than play clothes. English costume expert Doris Langley Moore recalled that in the 'teens "my mother, though by no means addicted to formality, would not allow us to appear beyond the confines of our own garden without gloves."[4] Though it is generally thought that American parents were less formal, it is doubtful that the children of upper–middle and wealthy families were allowed to dispense with this custom.

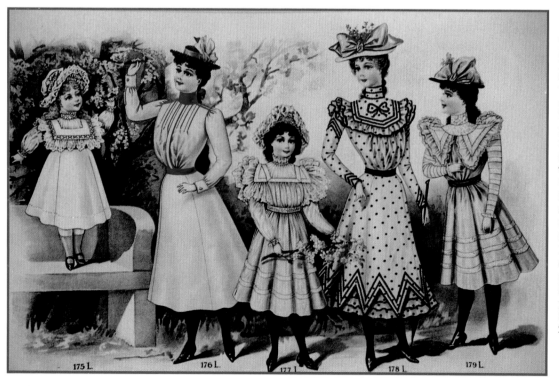

An 1899 *Delineator* fashion plate. *The Delineator* was published by Butterick sewing patterns, and therefore provided a fairly accurate view of what was being worn by the average person. Butterick's first magazine was *The Ladies Quarterly Review of Broadway Fashions*, published in the early 1870s. This was followed by *The Metropolitan Magazine* in 1877, and finally, *The Delineator* whose first printing numbered 10,000; by the turn of the century, many thousands more copies were printed, in addition to editions published in French, Spanish, and German. $25—$40.

175 L.     176 L.     177 L     178 L     179 L

## Facing The World

The first baby carriage was manufactured in England in the 1780s. Perhaps because it was created by a manufacturer of horse–drawn carriages, it (and all early baby carriages) was drawn or pulled by the child's nurse or mother, like a wagon. Nonetheless, by the early 1800s, the modern–style baby carriage (where the child was pushed instead of pulled) was beginning to be favored; the first American patent for such a carriage came in 1829.

There is little doubt that something like a baby carriage had been desired for many years. "The children in India are always carried by their nurses on a thickly–wadded cloth, consisting of many thicknesses of calico, run together, the edges trimmed with fringe," *Godey's Lady's Book* reported in 1857. "They are called *gooderies*. They afford a much more even and equitable surface for an infant's head and limbs to repose on than can be afforded by the arms of a nurse; and it is a pity, on every account, that the fashion is not adopted in this country."[1] The baby carriage had yet to become a nursery essential.

But that same year, construction began on New York City's Central Park, and by the end of the century, a park could be found in nearly every American town. These parks quickly became places where parents could promenade—and what better way was there to show–off an infant than with a baby carriage? Certainly a carriage was much more convenient than carrying the baby in arms, and because the design of the carriage could be excessively elaborate, there was ample opportunity for showy display. It wasn't until after World War One that baby carriages began to be designed less elaborately—and, significantly, that the child was situated so that he or she now faced the mother or nurse pushing the carriage, instead of facing the world.

[1] *Godey's Lady's Book,* 1857, p.362

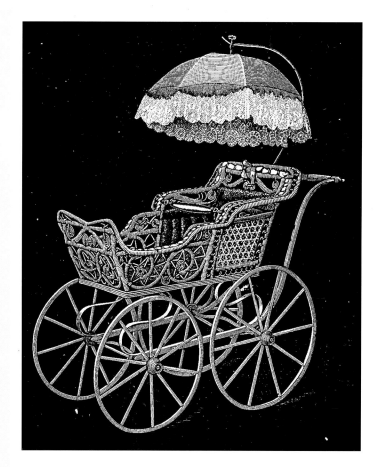

Baby carriages from the 1880s,
which originally sold for $15 to $30.

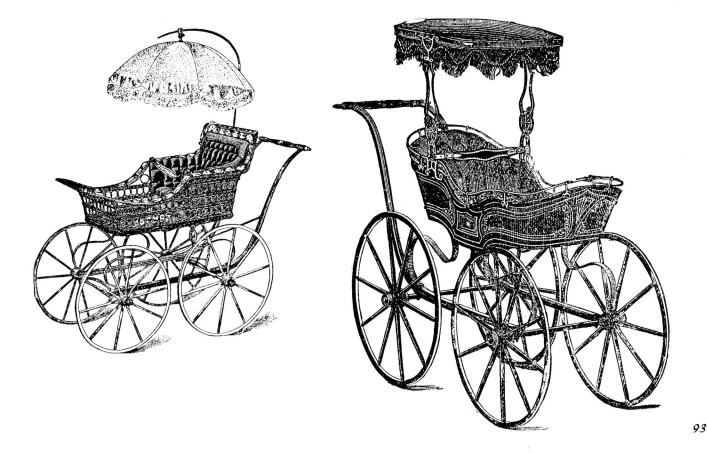

In both the 18th and 19th centuries, it was also customary for little girls to have their ears pierced. By the end of the 19th century, this had become an unusual custom—perhaps because of the flack it had received by certain influential writers, like Sarah Hale, editor of *Godey's Lady's Book*; she wrote and reprinted a fictional story (ending with a sermon) called "The First Ear-rings," several times for *Godey's*:

"'Dear me—Laura is eight years old to-day, and her ear-rings are not in yet!' exclaimed Miss Barbara Thorn, with great energy.

'But Aunt Barbara, she is only our baby yet, and pretty enough without ornaments, is she not?' said Mrs. Lucy Sellerman, the mother of little Laura, who had always trembled whenever her aunt alluded to the ear-rings...'Indeed, Aunt Barbara, I do think Laura is still too young to be tortured for fashion's sake...'

Poor little Laura! She stood supported by her gentle mother, who looked down on her daughter with that expression of love and sadness which marks the deep gush of the mother's heart, when the suffering, which she would so gladly bear for her child, can no longer be averted. How many hopes and fears rushed, like the changing colours of the evening sky, over the mother's mind, as she felt the pressure of Laura's little hands, and knew the dear child was stifling every expression of pain, lest it might distress her mother. 'At least,' thought Mrs. Sellerman, 'Laura is gaining self-control by this barbarous operation'...

Have any of the youthful readers of the *Lady's Book* a secret wish for jewels and costly ornaments? There are opportunities enough to display all these, without mutilating your flesh. Bracelets for the arms, rings for the fingers, necklaces and chains, pins and brooches of every description, and ornaments for the hair and headdress would seem sufficient to gratify the ingenuity and taste of those whose wealth or love of ornament leads them to study dress with a zeal amounting to passion...but the barbarous custom of mutilating the flesh, should not be encouraged by Christians. Let the fashion of boring the ears, in order to hand jewels therein, be left to the savages who wear rings in their noses to match; so we hope none of our young readers has an Aunt Barbara.[5]

Girls' hairstyles were also an important "fashion accessory." Though young boys were often subjected to the same torment of curls and hairbows, for them it ended at a much younger age—while for girls it never ended. A mass of curls has nearly always been fashionable for little girls, but never was the fashion so intense as at the close of the 19th and the opening of the 20th century. "They pay dearly for the glory of appearing in ringlets during the day if they are made to pass their nights laying upon a mass of hard rough bob [curlers]" one author of an etiquette book cried.[6] But most mothers chose a less torturous method of curling their daughter's hair—what we in the United States have traditionally called "rags:" Small sections of dampened hair were rolled onto thin strips of cloth, which were then knotted at the crown.

Curls were eminently important, but so were the bows that decorated them. In the 1890s, the fashion was usually for large floppy bows, but by 1900, the bow had shrunk considerably. That it was important to keep up with the latest trends in hairbows is testified to by many memories, including Gloria

Swanson's. "My maternal grandmother, who was in attendance [at my birth in 1899], leaned down to my pale, exhausted mother and said, 'She's beautiful.' Then she turned to the doctor, and lowering her voice so that her daughter wouldn't hear, asked, 'But aren't her ears awfully large?',", Swanson wrote. The effect of this attitude wasn't felt fully until she became old enough to have her hair styled. "While all the other girls my age were wearing teeny tiny hair ribbons," Swanson wrote, "my mother made giant silk bows and poufs for me to hide my ears."[7]

In all cases, however, it was the aim to teach girls to dress fastidiously, and to prepare them for the discomforts—but properness—of a woman's attire. "A girl's every-day toilet is a part of her character," *Happy Hours* magazine confided. "The maiden who is slovenly in the morning is not to be trusted, however fine she may look in the evening. No matter how humble your room may be, there are eight things it should contain: a mirror, washstand, water, soap, towel, hair, nail and tooth brushes. These are just as essential as your breakfast, before which you should make good use of them...Look tidy in the morning, and after the dinner work is over improve your toilet. Make it a rule of your daily life to 'dress up' for the afternoon. Your dress may, or need not be, anything better than calico; but with a ribbon or flower, or some bit of ornament, you can have an air of self-respect and satisfaction, that invariably comes with being well dressed. A girl with sensibilities cannot help feeling embarrassed and awkward in a ragged, dirty dress, with her hair unkept, if a stranger or neighbor should come in."[8]

Two articles of attire were worn by both young boys and young girls at the departure of the 19th century. One was the apron or pinafore—a tradition since the early 1800s, used to protect the clothes; while abandoned by boys in toddler-hood, girls continued to wear pinafores until puberty. The other garment worn by both boys and girls was the sailor suit.

The genesis of children's sailor suits seems to have come in 1846, when the five-year-old Prince of Wales (Prince Edward, later Edward VII), had his portrait painted in a sailor suit that he wore on the *Victoria & Albert* yacht on a royal visit to Ireland. This suit was, essentially, a scaled down version of a real-life navy uniform. Still, sailor suits were not widely worn by children until the 1880s, when, in the United States, the first publication of the official naval uniforms appeared—along with the introduction of four new, modern sailing ships with steam engines. The popularity of the sailor suit reached its peak in the 1890s, when the

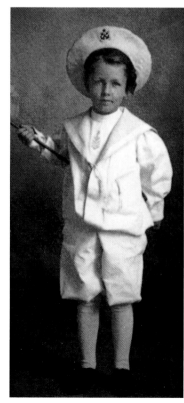

A boy from the turn of the century, wearing a classic "dressy" white sailor suit.

style became less of a miniature adult version, and more tailored to the child's body with knicker–pants and, often, short sleeves. Though navy was the most popular shade for sailor suits, white was worn on more formal occasions. "Sisters follow their brothers' example as nearly as they can in sailor suits," *The Lady's World* noted in 1887.[9] The only real difference was that girls wore a skirt instead of pants—though little boys not yet breeched also wore skirted sailor suits.

To compliment the sailor suit, sailor hats for both boys and girls were frequently worn. "Sailor hats of very coarse straw are stylish," *Godey's* noted as early as 1871. "For little boys they have no trimming but a piece of inch–wide ribbon velvet round the brim, short ends hanging at the back; sometimes blue and white or black and white striped ribbon replace[s] this. For little girls they often have a stiff wing, or aigrette, or feather tuft on one side."[10]

Though as late as the early 1900s, mothers could read that "petticoats for small boys are to be recommended in every way...the putting of infants at an early age into woolen knickerbocker suits cannot but be bad for them physically,"[11] more and more often, boys were being breeched at a very early age, wearing dresses only while infants. By 1900, shorts were fashionable, and by the late 1920s, it was unusual to see a boy—even an infant—in a dress. Still, there was a lingering effort to prevent children from behaving like children—to keep them inactive in order to keep them from spoiling their clothes. In 1905, *The Delineator* printed the following letter, typical in its motherly concern about this matter:

"I have a dear little boy who is very active. I am quite particular about his clothes, and he is so full of life I find it impossible to keep them looking clean and whole. I have punished him and find it of no use. He is in other respects a very obedient and affectionate child.

My friends say I am too indulgent with my little son; but it doesn't seem to spoil him, and it's always 'Mamma, dear,' and 'I love my mama,' and ever so many more little expressions of endearment for me. He is ever thoughtful of my welfare and so kind that I can't find it in my heart to deny him anything I can afford. Am I right in this? How should I act in regard to his clothes? I find it very hard to teach him to take care of them. He is only six years old, and I sometimes think I expect too much; but I admire a clean, wholesome–looking boy, and it's my ambition to have him so."

*The Delineator* answered this letter in a way that would have been radical only a few decades earlier—even though the revolution in children's wear had supposedly already occurred:

"It is impossible for the average child in the average environment to look spick and span all the time. Healthy, normal children delight in activity, and it is positively cruel continually to hamper their freedom by admonitions concerning the care of their clothing. Don't expect them to come in from play as clean as when they left the nursery, and don't, I beseech you, mothers, scold or punish them

A child's coat and a little girl's or boy's dress, from 1905.

when you see mud stains or an occasional rent. Look instead at the rosy, smiling faces and rejoice in the vitality and absence of self–consciousness, which are two of childhood's most precious possessions. Remember they cannot retain either of these in their pristine purity if they are constantly told to take care of the clothes or are received, after a morning's orgy with mud–pies or an hour in the brook, in some such fashion as this: 'Mercy me, Johnny, what a fright you are; you are mud from your head to your heels. Oh, don't come near me! Do not touch me! Why can't you keep yourself decent? I'm sure I never got so dirty when I was a child.'...

I should not punish a child for anything short of willful disregard of his clothing; for instance, if he should deliberately cut a piece out of a garment or commit some similar offense I should not mend the garment immediately, but have him wear it as it was, telling him I was sorry to see my little son with such a hole in his trousers, and the best way to make him remember not to do such a thing again would be to leave the hole so that he could see it. I should also say, after a day or so, that I would mend it as soon as he was quite sure he would *never, never* repeat the offense. Children who continue unduly heedless and who express no regret over the fact that their busy mother has to spend much time in mending the rents they make, might be dealt with in some–what the same way; but as you hope for lasting results in the training of your children and for harmony in your home, keep all your admonition free from any trace of resentment.

Since it should be our ambition to make the childhood of all children a period of such normal, wholesome activity and happiness that the memory of it will be a joy and inspiration to them throughout their lives, we can safely indulge all their reasonable wishes without fear of spoiling them...

Children should have some clothing especially adapted to play–hours, and in these garments they should be as free as air. If they are permitted this latitude they (continued, p.98)

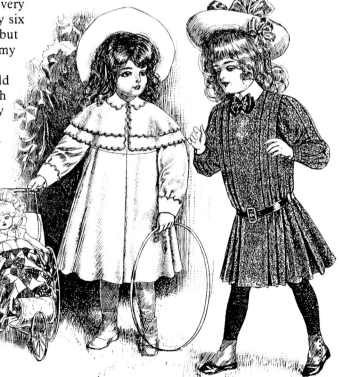

*The Craze For Fauntleroy*

No style of clothing has tormented little boys half as much as the Little Lord Fauntleroy styles of the late 19th century. Masculine memoirs are littered with sharp, ireful references to the style, which was based upon the drawings in Frances Hodgson Burnett's children's novel *Little Lord Fauntleroy*. Hodgson, an English–American, first wrote the story for American serialization in 1885, but boys did not feel the wrath of the fictional hero's influence until 1886, when Hodgson's story was published in book form in both the U.S. and England. The sentimental, patronizing novel was fantastically successful, selling over one million copies in England alone. Translated into over twelve languages, the novel earned the author over $100,000 while she was living, and after her death, earned her estate countless more. *Little Lord Fauntleroy* was also one of the first novels to be translated onto film—not to mention its success in various forms of theatrical plays.

As pictured in the accompanying illustrations by Reginald Birch, the hero Little Lord Fauntleroy was clothed in a black or deep royal blue velvet jacket with knickerbockers worn with a white blouse with a large lace collar (often referred to as a "Vandyke" collar, after the famous artist whose subjects inevitably wore large lace collars). A silk sash, silk stockings, buckled shoes, and shoulder–length, curled hair completed the outfit, which was based on one of Gainsborough's most famous paintings: the 18th century "Blue Boy," depicting a pre–teen in a fancy dress costume.

Little did the author and illustrator realize the misery they would be putting hundreds of little boys through.

"He started in life with a quantity of soft, fine, gold–colored hair, which curled up at the ends, and went into loose rings," Burnett described her young hero.

"He had big brown eyes and long eye–lashes and a darling little face. His manners were so good, for a baby, that it was delightful to make his acquaintance. When he was old enough to walk out with his nurse, wearing a short white kilt skirt, and a big white hat set back on his curly yellow hair, he was so handsome and strong and rosy that he attracted every one's attention, and his nurse would come home and tell his mamma stories of the ladies who had stopped their carriages to look at and speak to him. His childish soul was full of kindness and innocent feeling.[1]"

As romantic and charming as her description read, it inspired nothing less than revulsion from the children forced to wear the style pictured in the novel. Compton Mackenzie's response to the fashion is typical:

"That confounded Little Lord Fauntleroy craze which led to my being given as a party dress the Little Lord Fauntleroy costume of black velvet and Vandyke collar was a curse. The other boys at the dancing class were all in white [sailor] tops. Naturally the other boys were inclined to giggle at my black velvet, and after protesting in vain against being made to wear it I decided to make it unwearable by flinging myself down in the gutter on the way to the dancing class and cutting the breeches, and incidentally severely grazing my own knees. I also managed to tear the Vandyke collar. Thus not only did I avoid the dancing class, but I also avoided being photographed in that infernal get–up.[2]"

He was six years old when he wore the suit in 1889.

Even those who were not forced to wear the style by reason of their being too old to be dressed by their mother, complained bitterly of it. One gentleman wrote: "I saw a boy with a predestinate idiot of a mother, wearing a silk hat, ruffled shirt, silver–buckled shoes, kid gloves, cane, and a velvet suit with one two–inch pocket which is an insult to his sex."[3]

But to blame Burnett and Birch for putting countless young boys to shame isn't fair. In 1885 (a year before the illustrated *Little Lord Fauntleroy* appeared) the English magazine *The Lady* described a suit for "a little fellow of seven" consisting of a "tunic and knickerbockers of sapphire blue velvet and sash of pale pink. Vandyke collar and cuffs."[4] The novel's artist did not invent the style; the smashing success of the novel only put a stamp of approval on it, allowing fanciful mothers to indulge themselves.

Boys everywhere were thankful when the style was finally put to death in the early 'teens.

[1.] *Fabulous Century*, p.194.
[2.] *Children's Costume in England*, p. 187; *History of Children's Costume*, p.92.
[3.] *Men & Women*, p.149
[4.] *Children's Costume in England*, p.186–7.

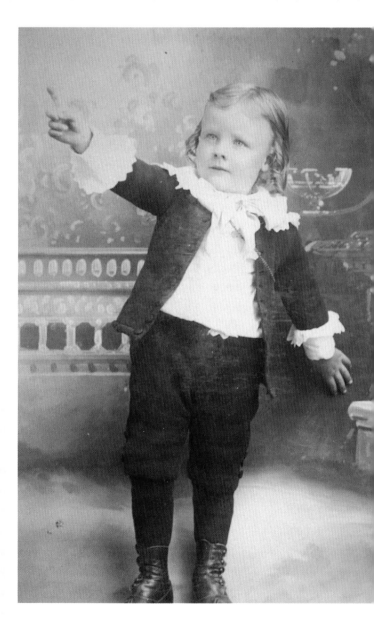

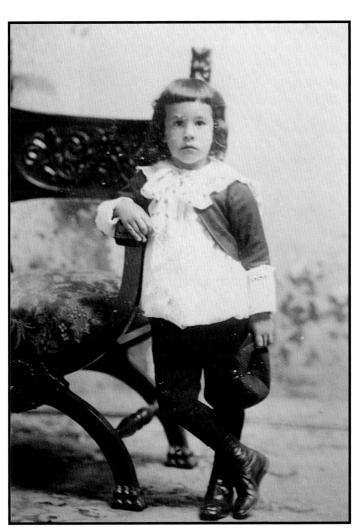

**Opposite page and left:** Two 19th century boys dressed in Fauntleroy style: ruffled shirts with wide, lacy, cuffs and collars, and tiny jackets.

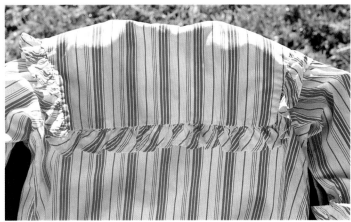

A perky "Little Lord Fauntleroy" style boy's shirt from the 1890s. *Courtesy of Antique Apparel.* $40—$70.

will, I assure you, take much more care of their best clothes at such times as it is right and proper for them to be this attired. I know a mother who from infancy impresses upon her children's minds the difference between their play clothes and their afternoon dresses. She tells them that papa likes them to have a grand good time in the morning, and doesn't mind in the least if they soil their clothes; but he likes to find them sweet and clean in the afternoon when he comes home, and so the afternoon amusements are of a quiet character—reading, story-telling, drawing, walking, quiet games, etc., etc., and habits of neatness are established without the enforcement of any irksome restrictions. Many a mother in this matter of children's apparel shows far more consideration for the imagined opinions of her friends and neighbors than she does for the comfort of the children.[12"]

The idea of clothes made and worn just for play, however, seems to have been only popular from the 1890s forward. Indeed, in the 18th century play was generally thought to be as waste of time, and something to be abandoned as soon as possible—age seven often being pointed to as a good age to end the unproductive time of play. "No more levity: childish toys and playthings must be thrown aside, and your mind directed to serious objects," Lord Chesterfield wrote to his son in the 1740s.[13] Rousseau, on the other hand, advocated play in large doses, and by the mid–19th century, play was more apt to be thought of as productive—*if* it was well directed.

"Boys and girls can learn many useful things in the guise of play," *McCall's* noted in the early 1900s. "Provide a place where they can have a bench and the necessary tools and show them how to make simple doll furniture. Give them a large packing box to turn into a doll's house. Teach them to stain the floors, paper the walls, make cheesecloth curtains, and shelves for the walls." But for girls the "play" advocated seemed less enjoyable: "All girls should learn how to sew, and one of the first practical lessons to be taught a home should be to make articles that are used in the household." Guides for mothers also advised a similar plan for play:

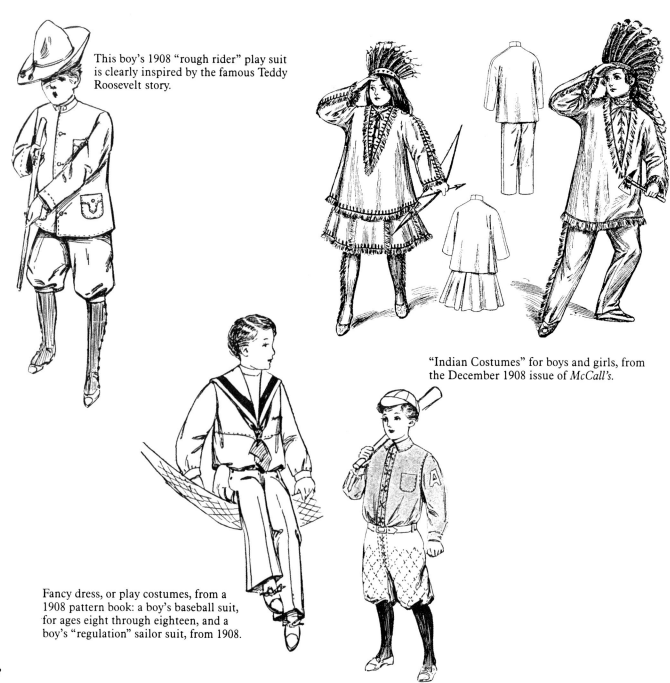

This boy's 1908 "rough rider" play suit is clearly inspired by the famous Teddy Roosevelt story.

"Indian Costumes" for boys and girls, from the December 1908 issue of *McCall's*.

Fancy dress, or play costumes, from a 1908 pattern book: a boy's baseball suit, for ages eight through eighteen, and a boy's "regulation" sailor suit, from 1908.

With wise direction the child will come to enjoy the work more than his play, and will gladly leave his romping if he can work with papa or mama...The girls may have miniature wash–tubs, wash–boards, flat–irons, pails, brooms, and brushes, and be taught how to use them. It is surprising how they will watch mother, and learn to imitate her. They can have needles and thread, scissors, and thimble, and be taught how to sew and darn. Their work will be imperfect at first, but it will rapidly improve under patient instruction.

If at all possible, provide a little shop for the boys, and give them a saw, hammer, and hatchet. Even with these tools, and a few nails and a pocket knife, you will be surprised and overjoyed to see what the little fellows make...There is nothing finer to interweave into a boy's education than the use of tools. They will teach him to think, to persevere, and to plan; and as he works, you will see that his mind is being drawn out and developed along the line of work at which he may be the most successful in after years.[14"]

Reading, too—much more than today—was a popular and desired sort of play. Though books for children were rare until the 1820s, there were a number of popular volumes that nearly every child owned if their parents could afford books. One was the English novel *The Governess*, written by Sarah Fielding in 1749. Though this book is virtually unknown today, another book, first published in 1812, is still a favorite among children: *Grimm's Fairy Tales*. Still, it wasn't until the 1860s that children's books meant for pure entertainment (though usually containing obvious morals) began to thrive.

Sets of cups, plates, and spoons were also often given to children as very practical toys. "Lovely bread and milk sets, consisting of plate, bowl, and pitcher, can now be bought for two dollars," *Good Housekeeping* noted in 1889. "Plates with the alphabet, or perhaps illustrating some fairy story, or maybe a geography lesson in the form of the map of the State in which the child lives, or some historical event pictured so as to tell a story," were frequently recommended as excellent ways to educate children in a fun way.

It really wasn't until the mid–19th century that toys as we think of them today were first manufactured; poorer children still relied on home–made toys, but the big business of toy–making was begun. Most toys were educational in some way; even dolls (probably the most–manufactured type of toy in the 18th, 19th and early 20th centuries) were considered educational, since they helped teach little girls how to be mothers. "I was absolutely mad for dolls," Gloria Swanson recalled. "I learned to walk by pushing a toy carriage with a baby doll in it...Later...I wouldn't even speak to other little girls if they didn't have babies of their own...I hated kindergarten from the first day for the simple reason that girls couldn't take their babies to school."[15] Paper dolls, also had an early existence, but reached their pinnacle of popularity when, in 1859, they evolved into ladies accompanied by various outfits of fashionable attire.

Precisely because dolls were considered a toy for teaching girls to be mothers, when the Teddy Bear was introduced in 1905, it created quite a stir. Inspired by the popular tale about President Theodore (Teddy) Roosevelt (who, the story goes, on a particular hunting trip could only find a bear cub, which he refused to kill), the Teddy Bear reached its peak of popularity in 1908, with millions sold in the United States. Manufacturers, however, often stressed that while it was a proper toy for a boy, it was inappropriate for his sister—the toy wasn't considered conductive to the maternal instinct.

Roosevelt's eldest daughter, Alice, recalled that as a well–off child in the 1880s her nursery was hardly littered with a wide variety of toys. Still, the choice of toys showed a distinct lack of sexism. "We used to have wonderfully made toys as children but not very many of them," she later recalled. "We had great bricks to build houses with. They used to come in large boxes which came by wagon. There were also windows and doors that came with them, but no glass. I also remember a firehouse that had scaled fire engines inside...There was a wonderful doll's house that belonged to my mother, and I used to play with that for hours. I also had my mother's doll with dresses done in the period when she was a child."[16]

The rocking horse, perhaps considered one of the most traditional toys of all, was another item that got off to a rocky start. In William P. Dewees' book (which was extremely popular in the early 1800s, and went through many editions), the idea was put forth that the rocking horse "should be considered a luxury, or it will be abused by becoming too familiar; it should, therefore, only be introduced occasionally, and that as a reward after good conduct."[17] The rocking horse may also have been subject to the same sort of opposition as the bicycle received in the 1880s and 90s. Not only were bicycles on the expensive side (an adult's version cost about $100), but they were suspected of degrading morals. The question was often raised whether girls and women should be given bikes, because, as one 1896 writer suggested, the seat of the bicycle might "beget or foster the habit of masterbation."[18]

## Endnotes:

1. *Ladies Home Journal*, Jan. 1895
2. *Children's Costume In England*, p.221
3. ibid., p.202
4. *Child In Fashion*, p.19
5. "The First Ear–Rings," *Godey's Lady's Book*, June 1843, p.253
6. *Miss Leslie's Behavior Book*, p.286–87
7. *Swanson*, p.13
8. *Happy Hours*, 1884
9. *Ladys' World*, 1887
10. *Godey's Lady's Book*, Dec. 1871, p.456
11. *History of Children's Costume*, p.129
12. *The Delineator*, Oct. 1905
13. *Martine's*, p.92
14. *McCall's*, Dec. 1908
15. *Swanson*, p.13
16. *Mrs. L.*, p.13
17. *Treatise on the Physical and Medical Treatment of Children*, 1825, p. 115
18. *Light of Home*, p.159

*Dressing for Make-Believe*

"There is nothing [a child] takes greater delight in than in imitation—playing somebody or something else," *McCall's* advised mothers in 1901.[1] But parents were seemingly slow to learn this. It wasn't until the mid–19th century that "fancy dress" or masquerade parties became popular past–times for children. As with many trends in the 19th century, Queen Victoria seems to have popularized the idea of children's costumes; she fancied dressing her own children up in whimsical or historical costumes, and then making watercolor sketches of them.

Yet in the 1850s, masquerades still had a scandalous taint to them, and memories of wild 18th century fancy dress parties still lingered. "The expediency of children's parties is a question not yet at rest by the magazines and journals devoted to nursery tactics," *Godey's Lady's Book* said in 1850. But children's strong longing for make–believe was winning out. "In the mean time," the editors wrote, "children will enjoy themselves after this fashion, and as there are mothers indulgent enough to gratify them, we give a plate of some of the prettiest costumes Parisian taste and elegance have copied or invented...The costumes, though, at first sight, seeming so costly, can be easily arranged at very little expense. Any mother with ordinary taste and ingenuity, could do so with a few purchases; and, as the dress is worn but once or twice at most, there is not much matter about the length of stitches. Indeed, a very pretty costume has been finished with the aid of pins alone."[2]

Soon, fashion magazines began touting the idea that masquerade costumes could actually prove beneficial to children—not only were they fun to play in, but they could educated their little wearers, as well. Often this "education" was strongly founded in history. Author Lewis Carrol described one 1875 English fancy dress party where history was ever–present: "I came yesterday, to be present at a children's fancy ball, which was a very pretty sight. The house is Elizabethan, so most of the dresses were of that period, the eldest girl, Maud, being dressed as Queen Elizabeth, and the ball began with a grand royal procession, which was very well done."[3]

Yet by the 1880s, fancy dress was not just for wealthy children; old clothes were often re–made into costumes, which could be as simple as splashing an old, tired dress with ink to make it appear spotted. In fact, children's fancy dress was becoming more popular than adult fancy dress, and in England, sewing pattern publishers issued magazines consisting entirely of children's fancy dress patterns.[4] Typically, the child's fancy dress costume was as elaborate as his or her parents' could afford, but in the 1920, a revolution took place. Cheapness was now the key to a good costume, and crepe paper costumes became vogue. The new fancy dress costumes were less historical, and more playful—even commercial. Nonetheless, magazines continued to tout the educational value of make–believe:

"Mothers can do much to keep their little ones [out of trouble] by encouraging the right kind of play...What child would not be wild with joy to possess [this Indian] suit? Think of the Wild West shows they could give, the wonderful games they could improvise. A brood of little ones, a tent in the back yard and a few such suits, and there will be no end of fun in that back yard and blissful quiet in the house. And, again, what little boy or girl has not been invited to a masquerade or fancy dress party? Here would be an opportunity to inspire the wildest admiration among the small guests, for all the child world loves a brave warrior. A Christmas gift of this kind would mean much more to a child than some of the meaningless and fragile toys, of which he soon tires. There is no trouble, and but small expense, attached to the making of this suit...The suit can be made up for a boy or girl, as the pattern provides both skirt and trousers....A little ingenuity and an abundance of chicken feathers will contribute greatly to the warlike fierceness of the Indian brave's head–dress. Pochontas, being a very amiable little squaw, will be satisfied with the smaller quantity of feathers.[5]

[1.] *McCall's*, Dec. 1908, p.26
[2.] *Godey's Lady's Book*, Jan. 1850
[3.] *Fancy Dress*, p.27
[4.] *Child In Fashion*, p.80
[5.] *McCall's*, Dec. 1908, p.26

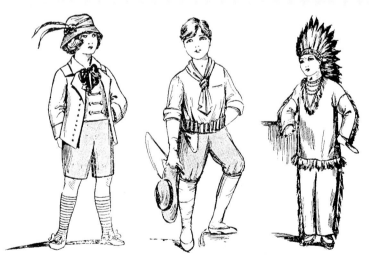
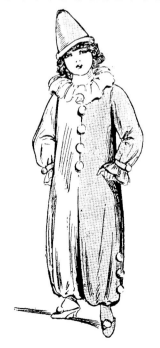
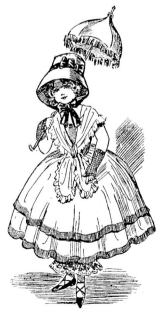

Fancy dress costumes, from the 1913 *Young Ladies' Journal Extra Christmas Number*. Featured are costumes for a "Tyrolese Peasant," a "Cowboy," a "Red Indian," a "French Clown," and an "Early Victorian."

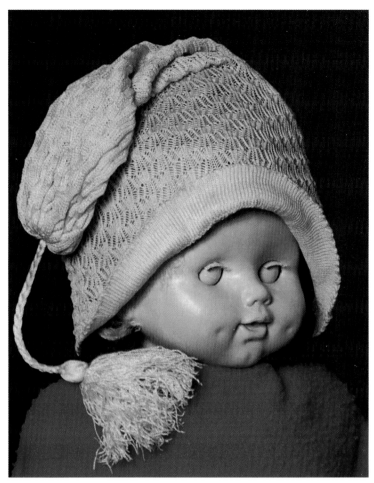

A hand made baby's cap featuring a long tassel, c.1890–1915. *Courtesy of Persona Vintage Clothing.* $10—$35.

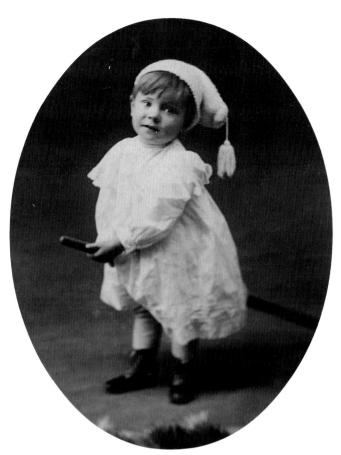

A boy from the turn of the century wearing a similar cap. He also dons a white dress trimmed with tucks and lace.

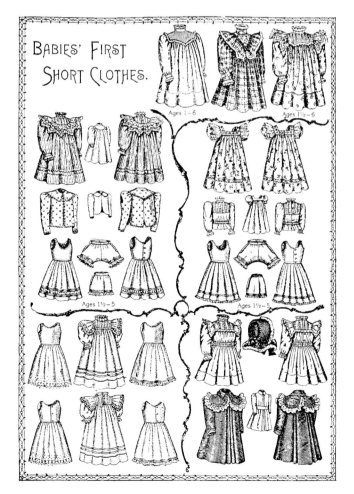

*The Delineator* featured these "essential" sets of baby's clothes in 1899.

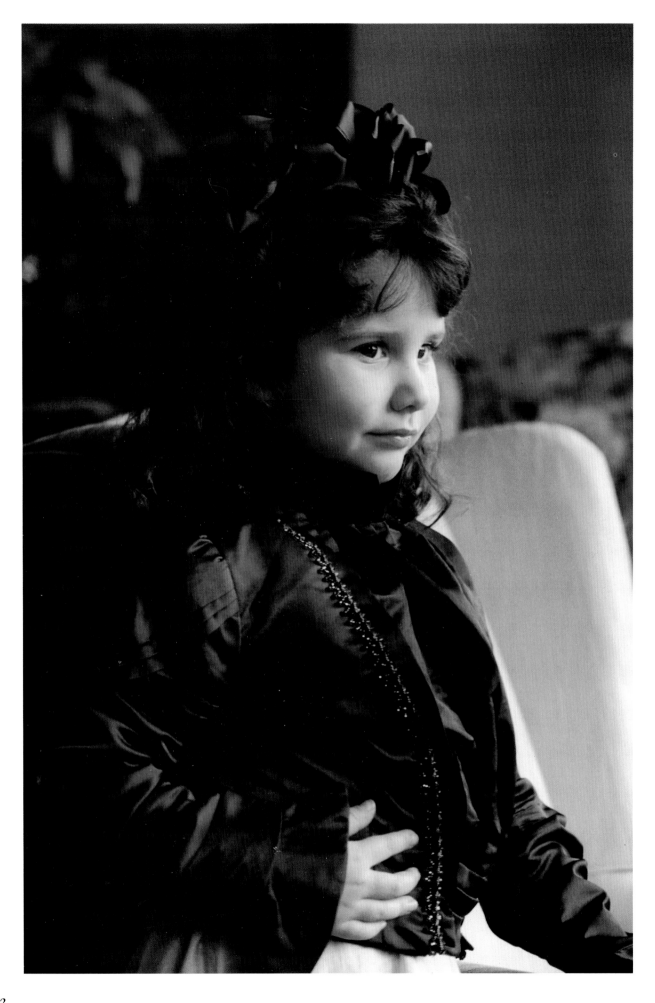

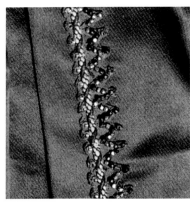

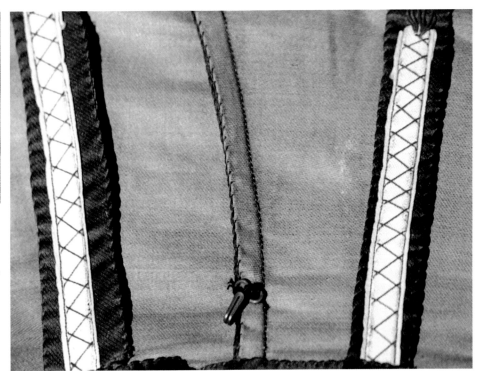

Opposite page, above and right:
This c.1899–1904 girl's silk bodice features magnificent beading. The inside is boned, just as an adult woman's bodice would be. *Courtesy of Vintage Silhouettes.* $50—$75.

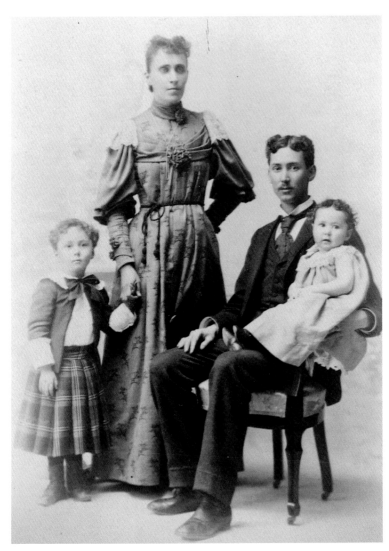

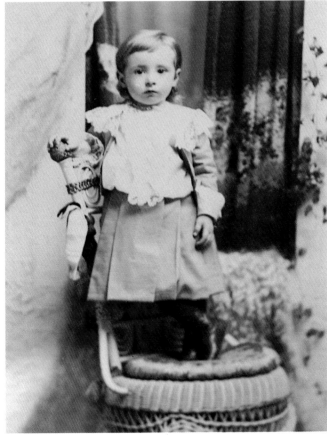

By the 1890s, boys were generally being breeched at an earlier age, but the tradition of boys' dresses died slowly, as these photos from the 1890s illustrate.

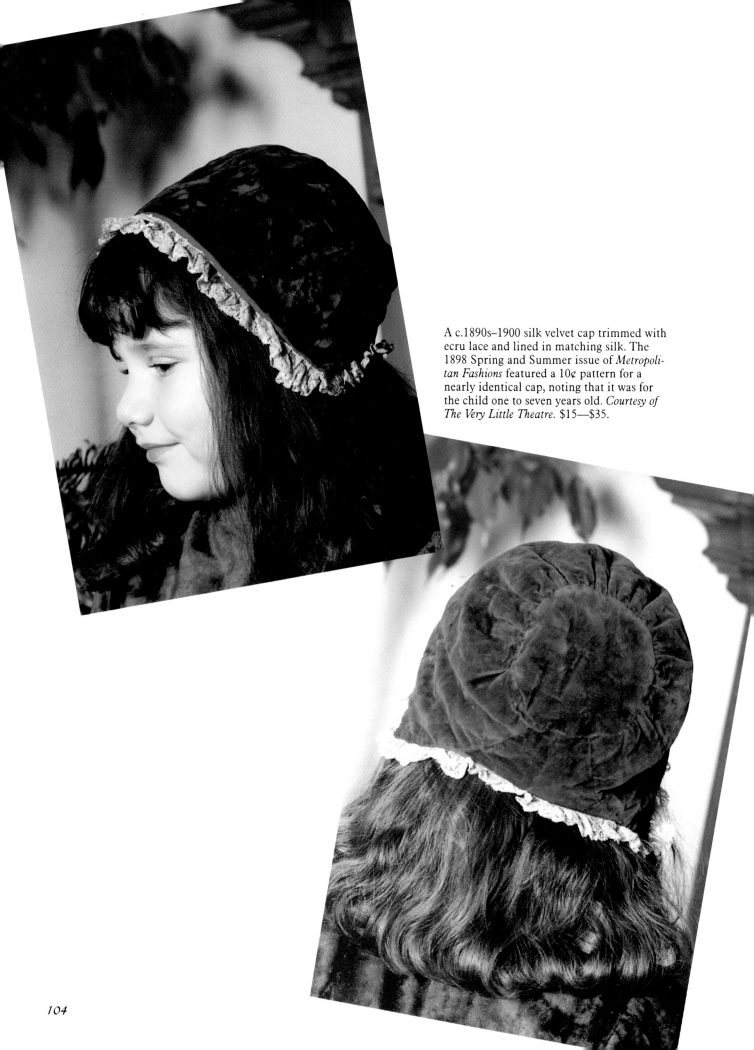

A c.1890s–1900 silk velvet cap trimmed with ecru lace and lined in matching silk. The 1898 Spring and Summer issue of *Metropolitan Fashions* featured a 10¢ pattern for a nearly identical cap, noting that it was for the child one to seven years old. *Courtesy of The Very Little Theatre.* $15—$35.

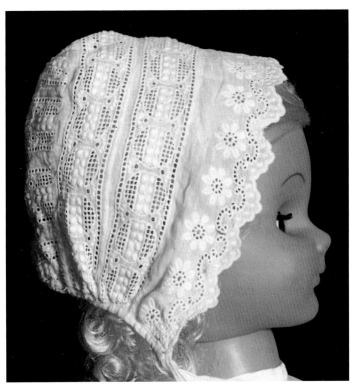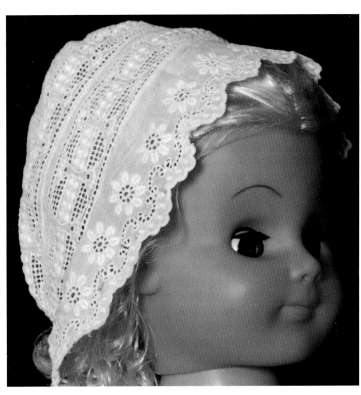

A typical infant's cap from the turn of the century, fashioned out of eyelet. $5—$15.

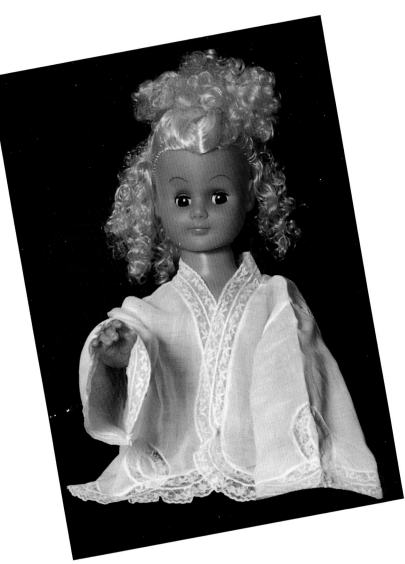

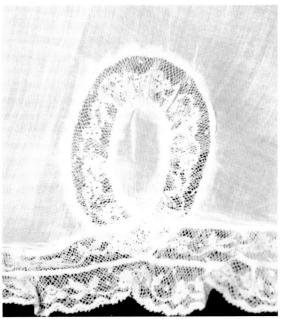

A c.late 1890s—'teens baby's kimono of cotton with extensive lace insertion. It is entirely open in front, with no closures. *Courtesy of The Very Little Theatre.* $20—$45.

Typical baby layettes, from 1899.

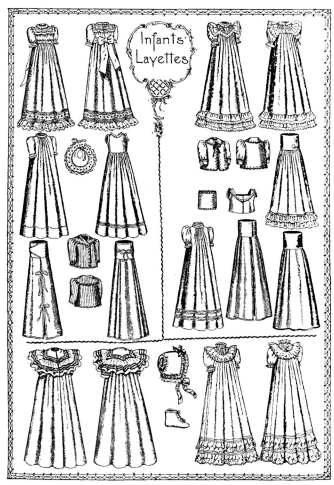

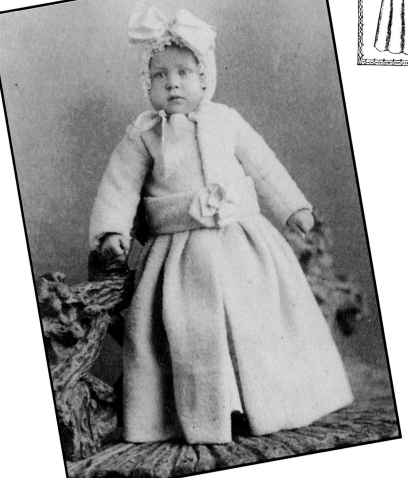

Reminiscent of the nursery rhyme about baby bunting, this baby, photographed in the 1890s, is snugly wrapped in a jacket/dress and bonnet.

**Opposite page:** A c.1898–1900 girl's dress of velvet. The gored skirt is fitted onto a 1/2 inch waistband; the yolked bodice features a 1/2 inch high collar and is slightly pigeon–fronted. The dress closes with hooks and eyes down the back. Fashion magazines of the period rarely featured such simple girl's dresses. $90—$125.

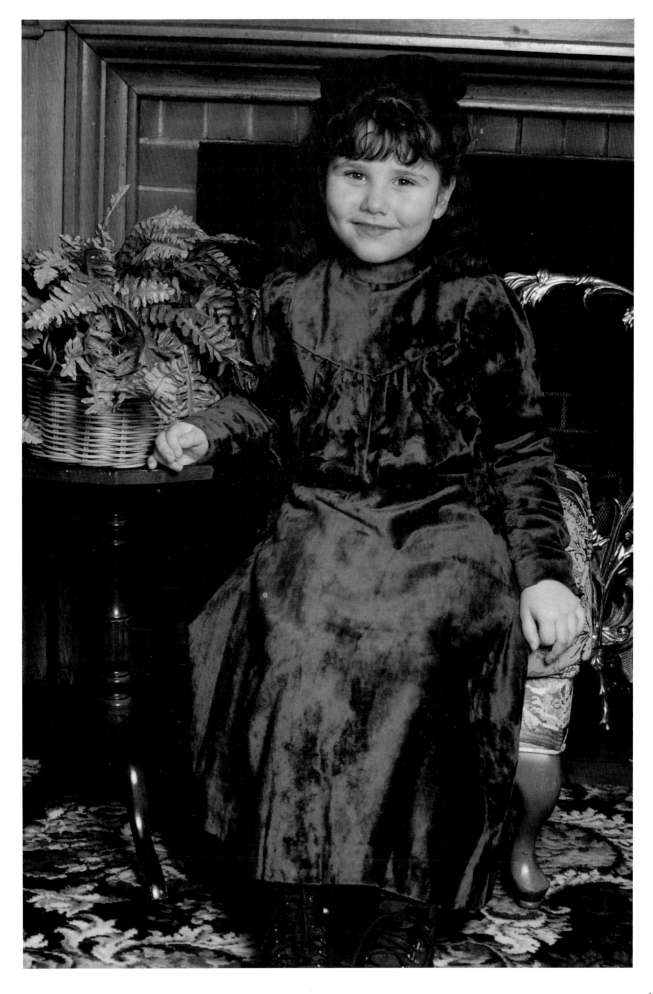

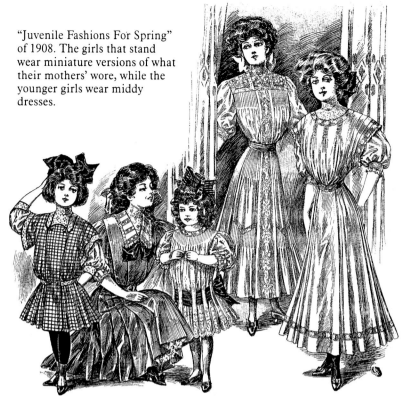

"Juvenile Fashions For Spring" of 1908. The girls that stand wear miniature versions of what their mothers' wore, while the younger girls wear middy dresses.

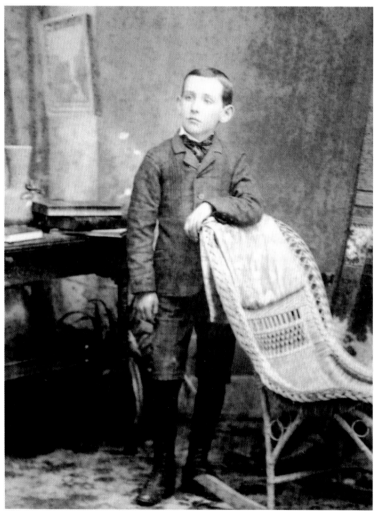

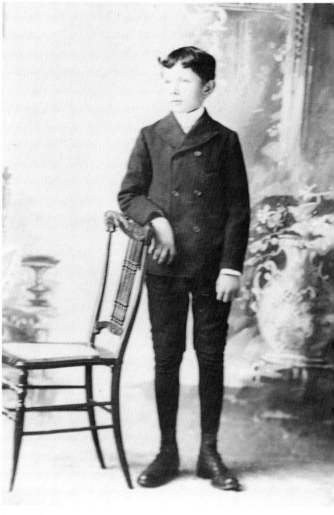

Two young lads from the 1890s, wearing knickered suits.

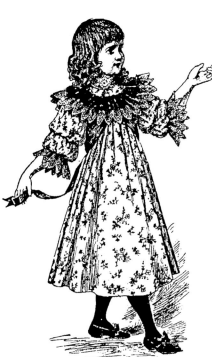

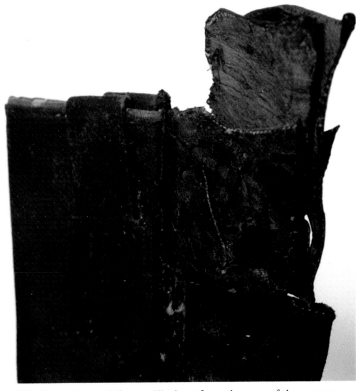

A boy's cowboy or infantry–like boot from the turn of the century. *Courtesy Antique Apparel.* $85—$125.

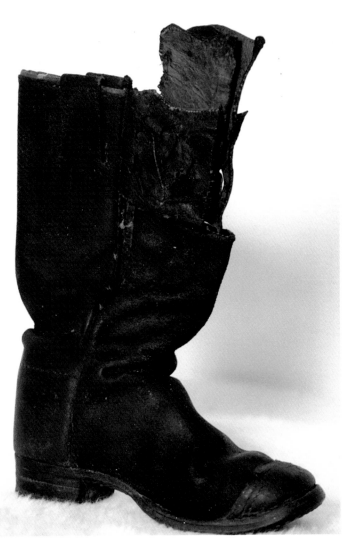

In the 1890s, the high–waist empire style that had been popular in the early 1800s was revived for both women and children. These two empire dresses were featured in a dressmaker's magazine: the plain one in 1895, and the patterned one in 1893.

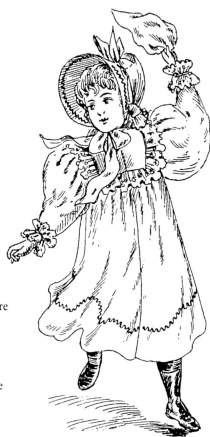

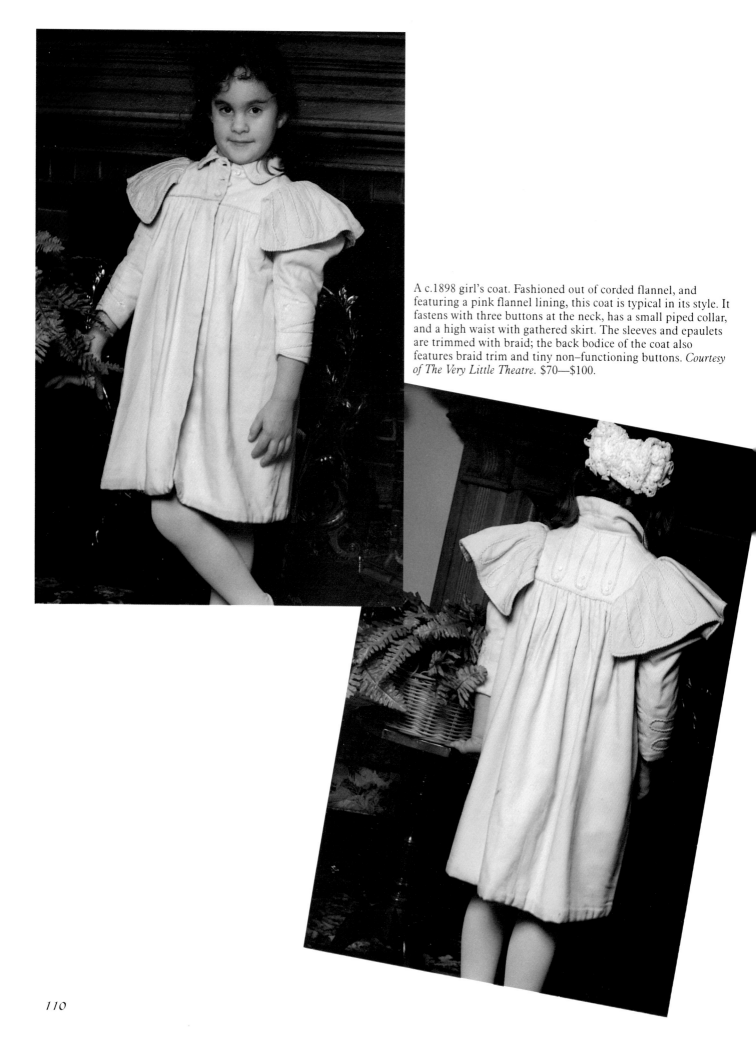

A c.1898 girl's coat. Fashioned out of corded flannel, and featuring a pink flannel lining, this coat is typical in its style. It fastens with three buttons at the neck, has a small piped collar, and a high waist with gathered skirt. The sleeves and epaulets are trimmed with braid; the back bodice of the coat also features braid trim and tiny non–functioning buttons. *Courtesy of The Very Little Theatre.* $70—$100.

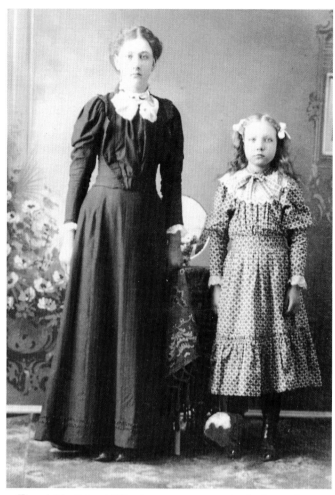

The girl in this c.1890s photo wears a very basic dress—but one that has many fashionable elements. The two–piece sleeve is typical of this date, as is the puffed bodice front.

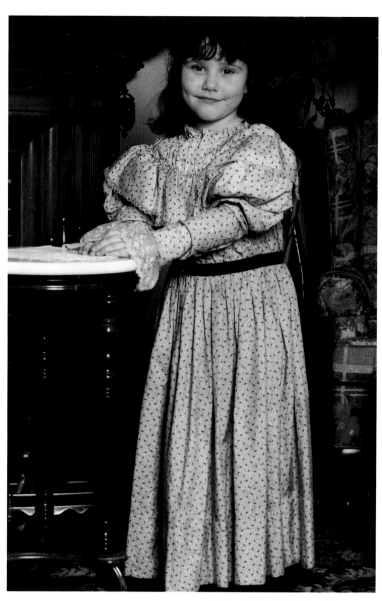

This c.1898 girl's dress is fashioned out of a printed silk. The yolk is shirred and trimmed with lace, and the two–piece sleeve (full at top, slim at bottom) ends with a frill of lace. A black silk ribbon adorns the waistband. *Courtesy of The Very Little Theatre.* $100—$200.

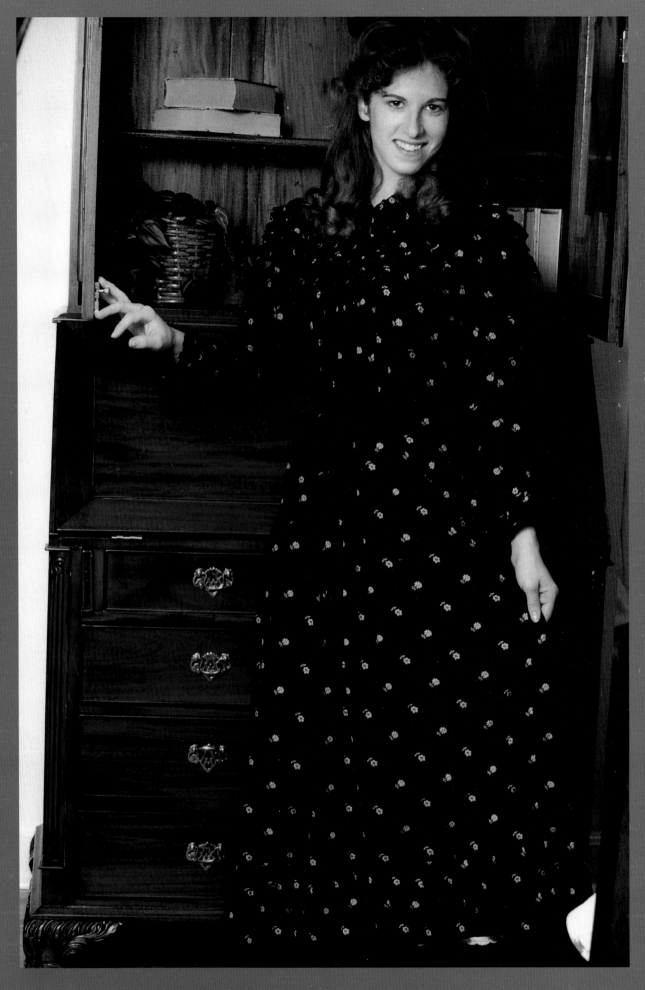

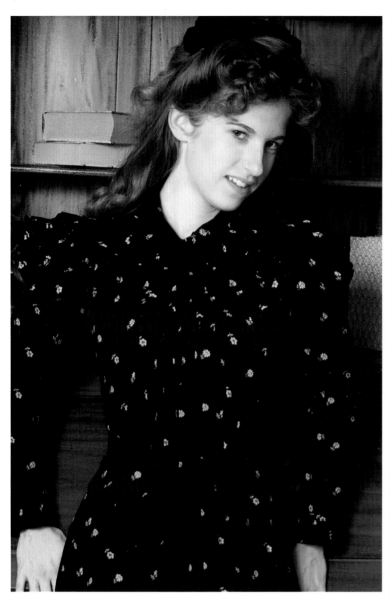

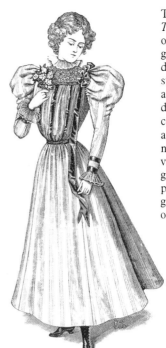

The March 1897 issue of *The Standard Designer* offered the pattern for this girl's dress for 20¢. It was described as "simple in style, but very *chic* in appearance. The pattern is developed in striped rose–colored lawn, with lace yolk and white chiffon ruffle for neck and wrists. Cerise velvet ribbon is used for girdle and decoration." The pattern was available for girls ten to sixteen years old.

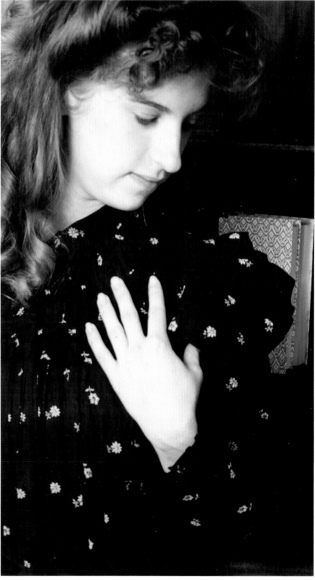

**Opposite page, above and right:** This young misses' cotton wrapper or tea gown dates to c.1890–1905. Wrappers were worn only in the house and amid family and close female friends for breakfast, tea, or in preparation for an evening's outing. They were intended to be comfortable but neat, and though this wrapper appears to close only with a ribbon tie around the waist, it has a fitted inner bodice that buttons up the front. An 1894 Montgomery Ward catalog featured a similar wrapper for $1.45. *Courtesy of Vintage Silhouettes.* $125—$225.

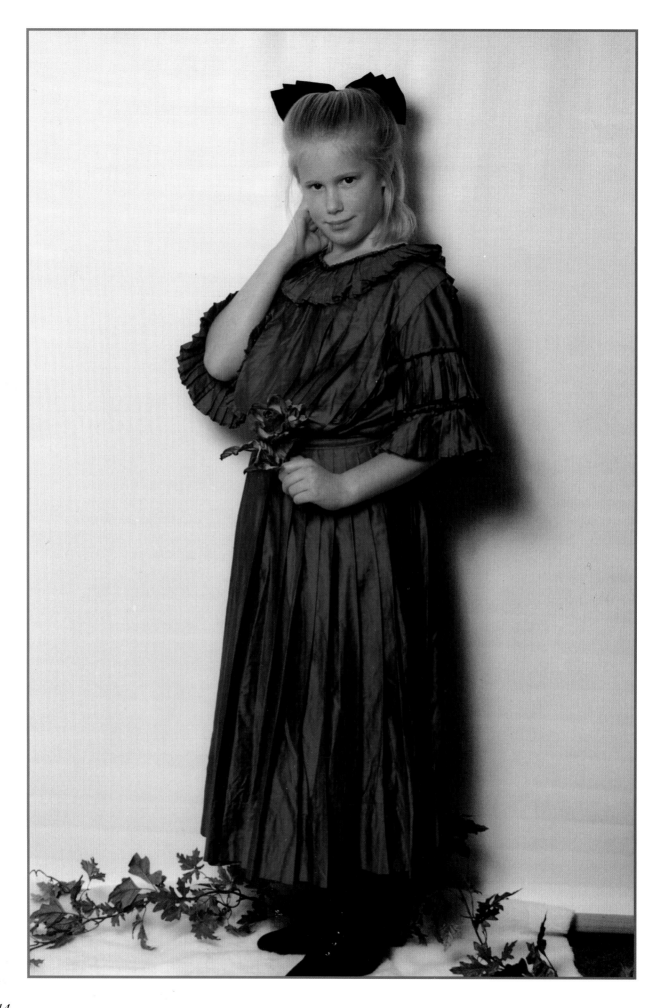

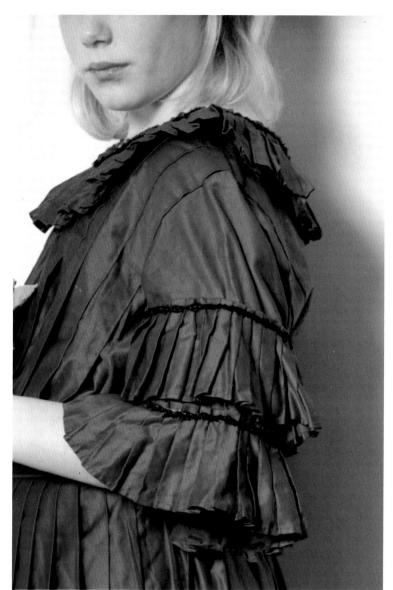

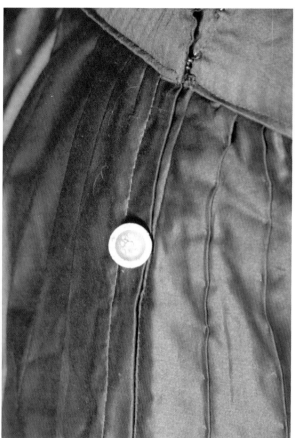

**Opposite page, left and above:** A special–occasion dress for a young miss, c.1890–1900. Fashioned out of a stunning raspberry cotton/silk blend, the dress features a rounded neckline trimmed with a ruffle and a string of jet. The pleated bodice and short sleeves are trimmed with jet and two pleated ruffles. Though buttons are sewn to the back of the dress, they are non–functional; the dress closes in back with hooks and eyes. A separate matching petticoat of the same fabric is worn under the dress. *Courtesy of Vintage Silhouettes.* $200—$350.

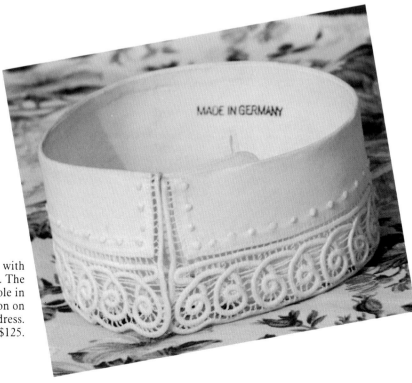

A rare girl's paper collar, c.1890—1910 with extensive hand embroidery and faggoting. The collar buttons in front, and has a buttonhole in back that would correspond with the button on the back neckline of a shirtwaist or dress. $95—$125.

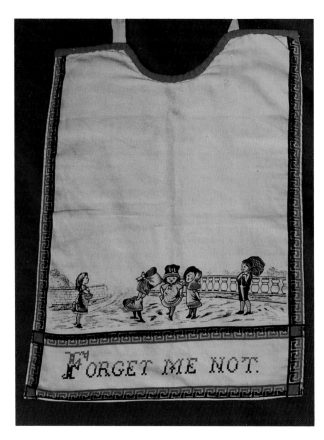

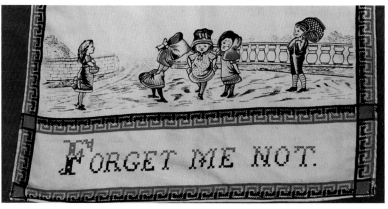

This printed bib seems to show some influence from Kate Greenaway's drawings, and is probably c.1890–1903. It measures approximately 10 inches wide by 13.5 inches long. *Courtesy of Pam Coghlan.* $100—$185.

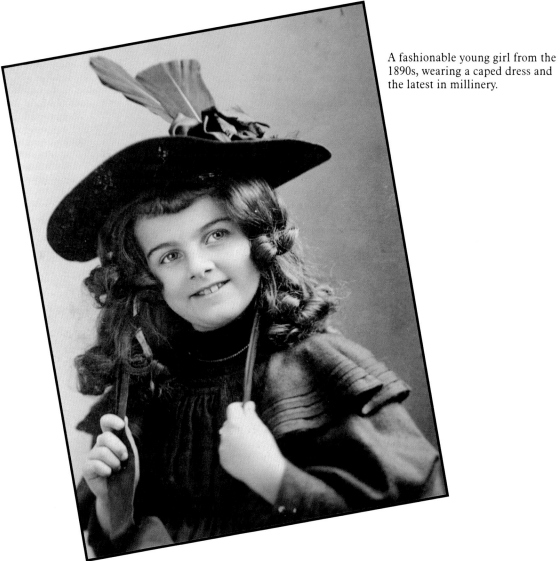

A fashionable young girl from the 1890s, wearing a caped dress and the latest in millinery.

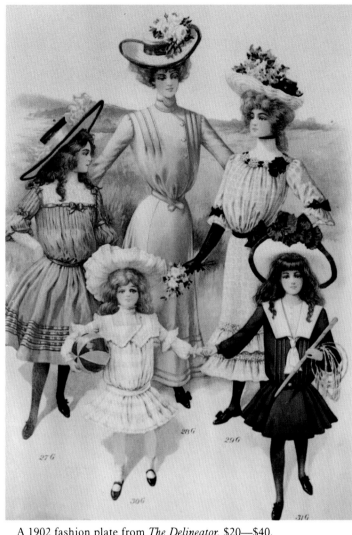

A 1902 fashion plate from *The Delineator*. $20—$40.

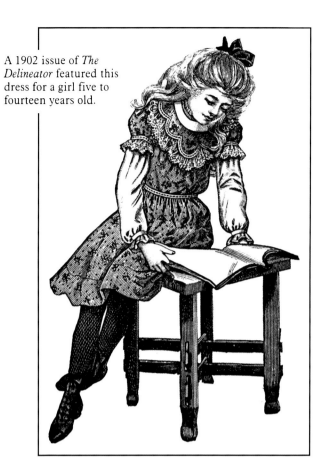

A 1902 issue of *The Delineator* featured this dress for a girl five to fourteen years old.

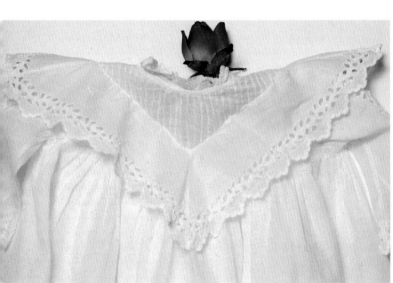

A c. 1900–1910 christening gown of cotton, 31 inches in length. The V-shaped yolk trimmed with pintucks and a flounce was very up to date. Two tiny, hand crochet buttons close the gown in back. $60—$95.

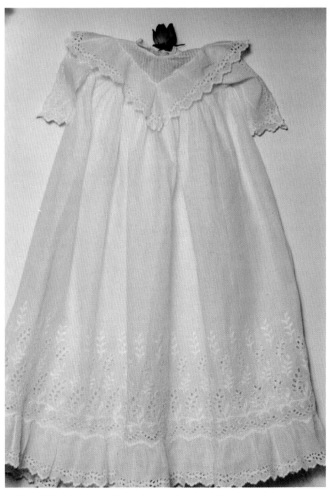

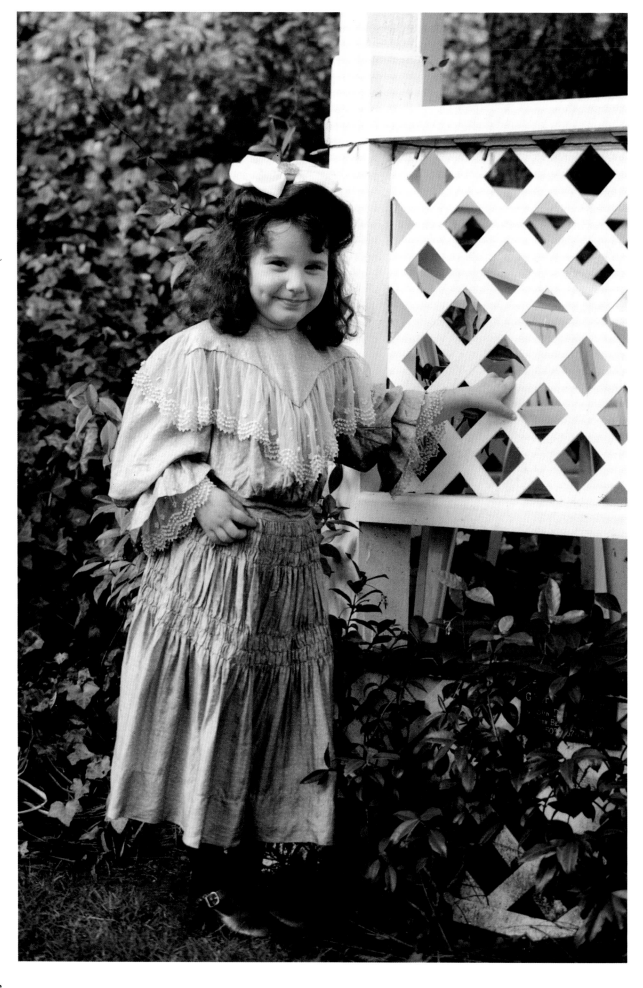

A girl's c.1900–05 dress of blue silk specked with white. The V–shaped yolk is lavishly trimmed with a wide gathered flounce of lace, also found at the sleeve cuffs. The skirt is heavy smocked, and hooks and eyes close the dress down the back. *Courtesy of Vintage Silhouettes*. $125—$300.

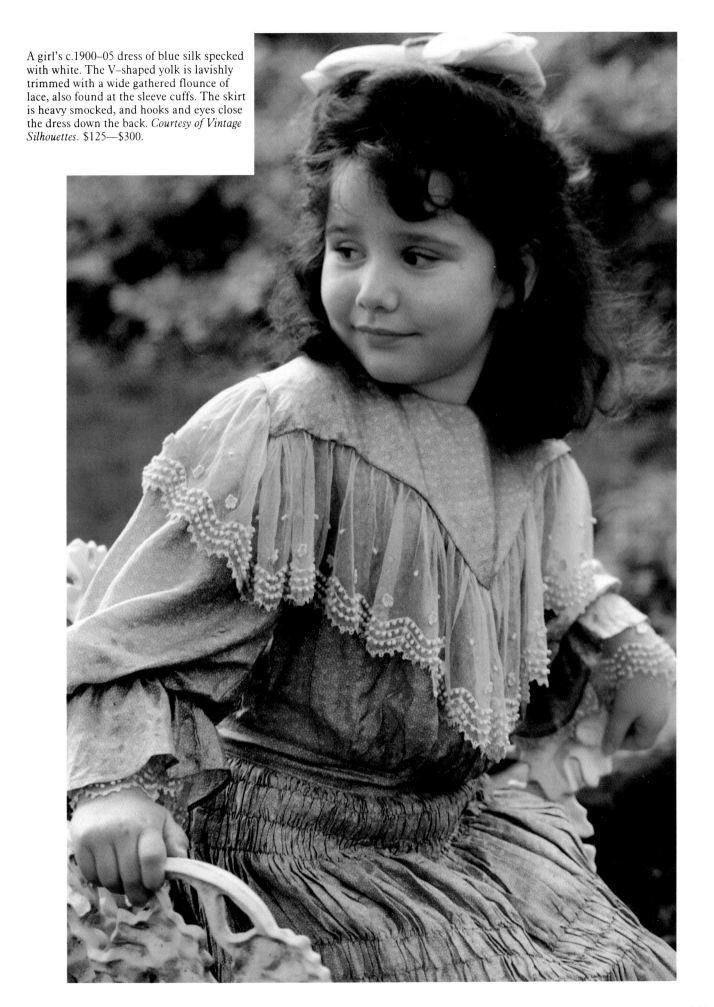

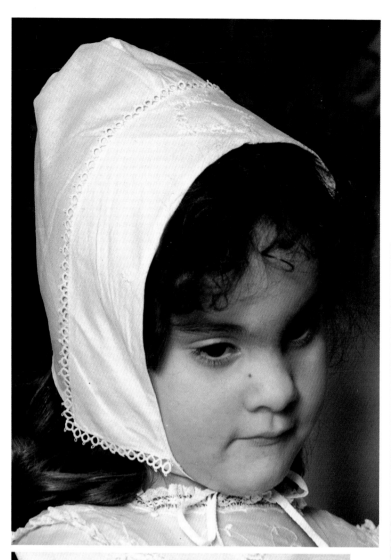

**Opposite page:** A turn of the century portrait of siblings. The child on the right wears a Little Lord Fauntleroy–inspired ruffled shirt, while the child on the left wears a pure white, crochet–trimmed dress.

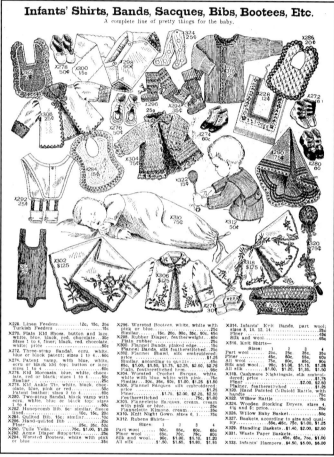

A turn of the century Lipman, Wolfe, & Co. catalog featured this page of ready–made infant goodies, ranging from bibs and stockings to diaper supporters and shoes, costing between 10¢ and $6.

A c.1900–1915 Dutch–style bonnet; the turned–back brim is trimmed with whitework and crochet. *Courtesy of The Very Little Theatre.* $5—$15.

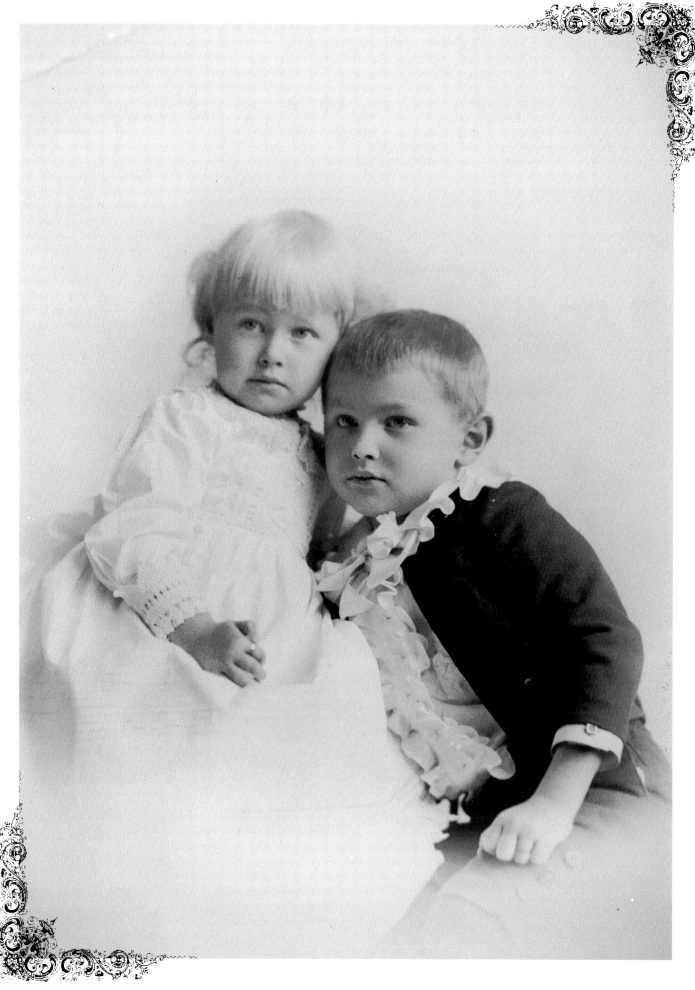

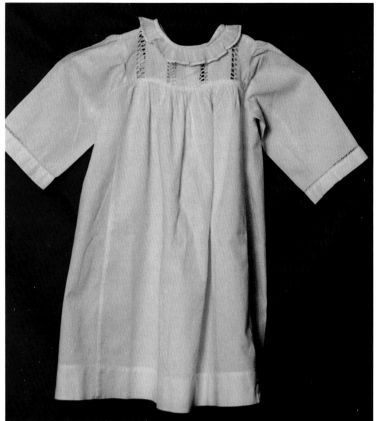

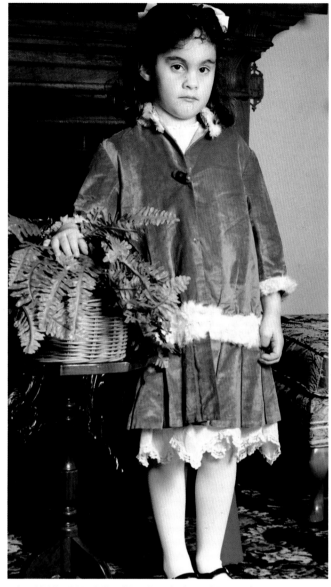

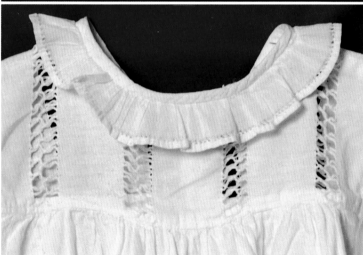

A c.1905–1919 baby's dress featuring extensive faggoting. *Courtesy of The Very Little Theatre.* $10—$40.

A c.1905–1909 girl's silk velvet jacket with real fur accents. It closes in front with snaps; the single oblong celluloid button is a "faux" closure. *Courtesy of The Very Little Theatre.* $70—$95

A baby's petticoat dating to the late 19th or early 20th century. Like adult petticoats of the period, it is well trimmed with eyelet and tucks. The petticoat opens at one side and has five buttonholes on waistband, which would have been used to button the petticoat onto a corset or chemise. *Courtesy of Amazing Lace.* $24—$45.

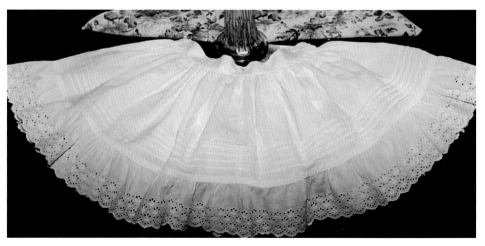

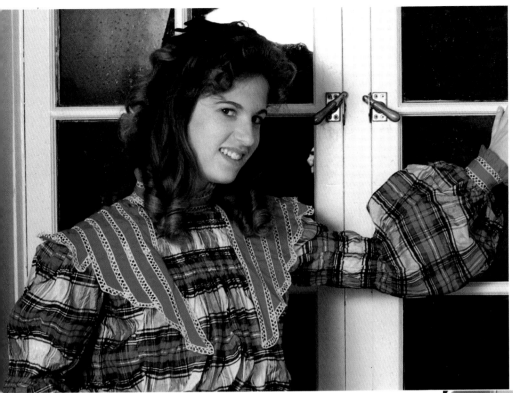

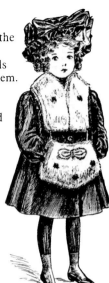

Furs of all kinds were not entirely the domain of grown women. Little girls also often wore them. This child's set consisting of an ermine muff lined in silk, and a matching ermine neckpiece, was designed for a child under six, and sold for a mere 50¢.

A c.1900–05 red silk plaid young misses' dress with a stunning solid red collar, epaulets, cuffs, and waist ribbon. The smocked bodice is fastened with hooks and eyes down the back. Three short bones are sewn to the center back of the bodice. *Courtesy of Vintage Silhouettes.* $185—$400.

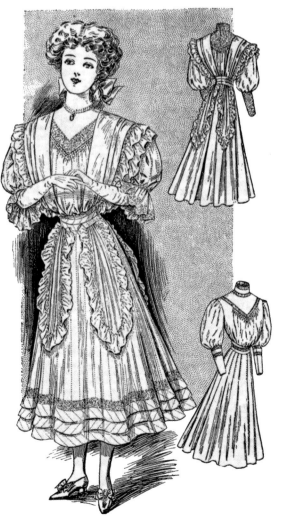

A dress for a thirteen to seventeen year old girl, as featured in an April 1908 issue of *McCall's*.

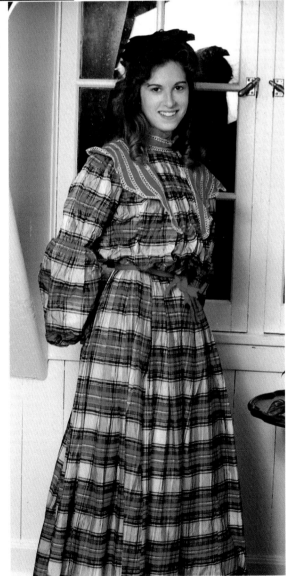

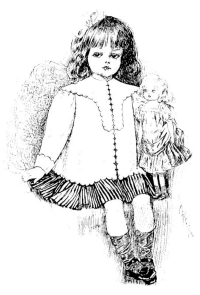

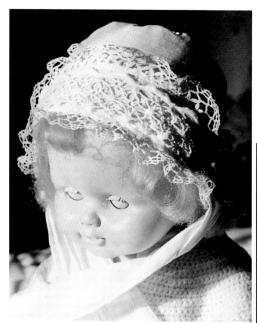

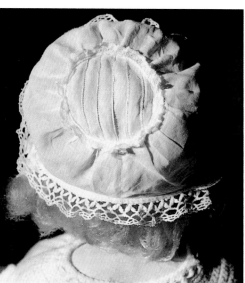

This baby's cap dates to the early 1900s, and is trimmed with hand crochet. *Courtesy of Persona Vintage Clothing.* $25—$35.

*The Delineator* featured this child's "house–sack" in October of 1905, and sold the pattern for a five to seven year old for 10¢. The editors pointed out that it was important to have "dainty and useful little garments for wear indoors in the cool Autumn days."

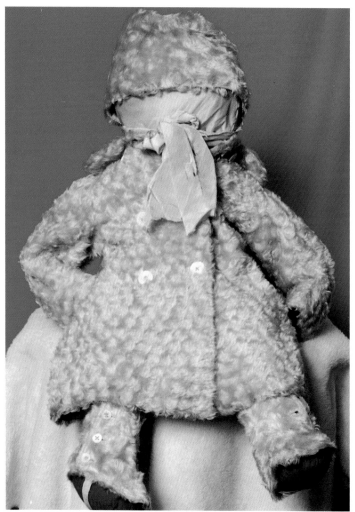

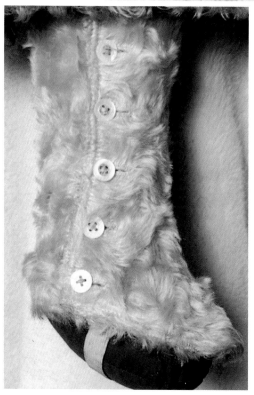

A remarkable three–piece mohair "teddy bear" suit, c.1907–1915. The double–breasted coat has cuffed sleeves, and the separate leggings each have 11 buttons running down the side and an elastic strap for the foot. The cap ties with silk ribbon; each piece of this ensemble is lined with cream–colored cotton. Teddy bear items of all sorts (from pillows to paper dolls) were the rage by 1908, a year after they were introduced; Sears catalog from that year featured a variety of teddy bear items, with the note that the teddy bear was "not a fad or campaign article, but something which has come to stay on merit alone." *Courtesy of Pam Coghlan.* $250—$400.

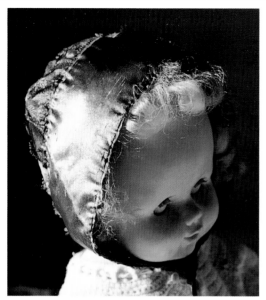

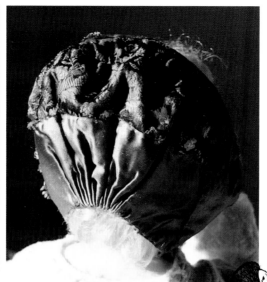

A baby's bonnet from the estate of a Scandinavian immigrant family. Dating to the early 1900s, the bonnet is fashioned out of a silk print and silk solid, and is garnished with self fringe. *Courtesy of Persona Vintage Clothing.* $15—$25.

Clearly inspired by Kate Greenaway and the fashions of the early 19th century, this girl's bonnet was featured in an 1905 issue of *The Delineator.* The editors described it as "a quaint little bonnet that will be very attractive on a wee maiden."

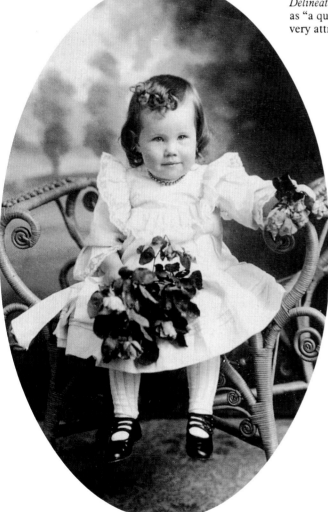

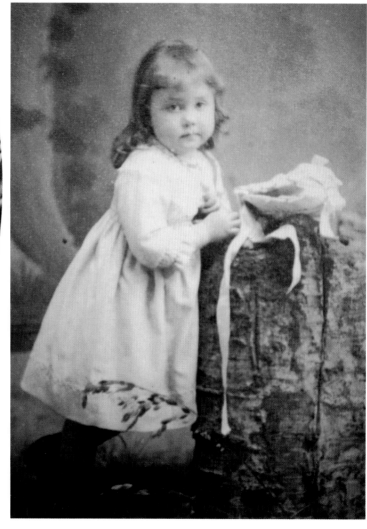

Little white dresses, so popular at the beginning of the 19th century, were once again the rage at the beginning of the 20th century.

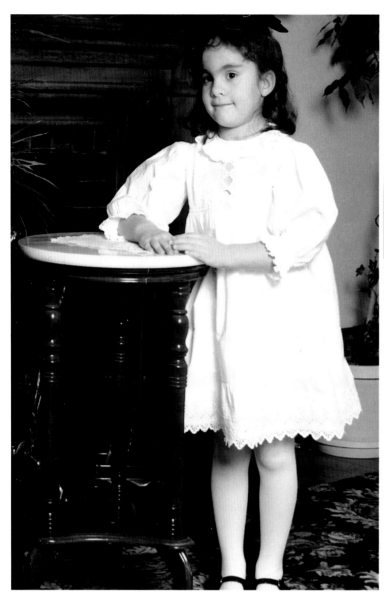

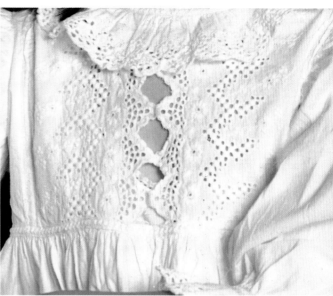

A c.1900–1909 toddler's dress with a round, gathered eyelet collar and a yolk composed of eyelet. The sleeves are puffed and end in ruffle of eyelet; the hem is also trimmed with eyelet. *Courtesy of The Very Little Theatre.* $20—$40.

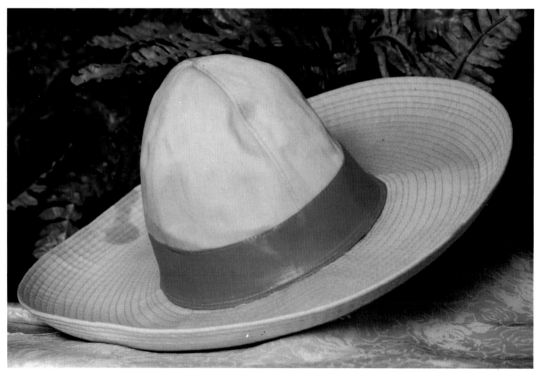

A boy's Teddy Roosevelt–style hat, c.1901–1919. A 1918 Sears catalog illustrated a "Military Outfit" for boy, which featured a similar hat. *Courtesy of Vintage Silhouettes.* $30—$45.

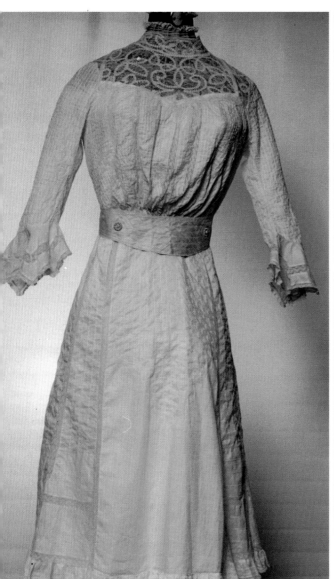

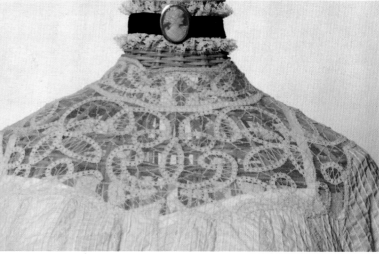

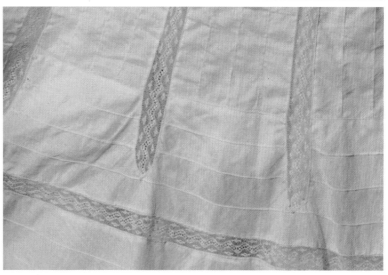

This cotton c.1900–1903 girl's dress is entirely composed of pintucking and lace insertion, with a bodice yolk of net work. Eight tiny 1/4 inch buttons close the bodice in back. *Courtesy of Mother & Daughter Vintage.* $150—$250.

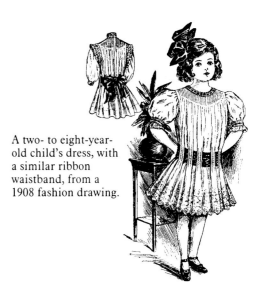

A two- to eight-year-old child's dress, with a similar ribbon waistband, from a 1908 fashion drawing.

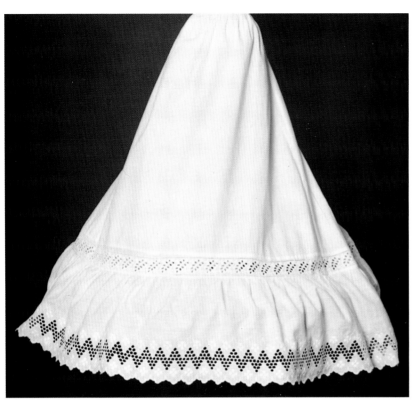

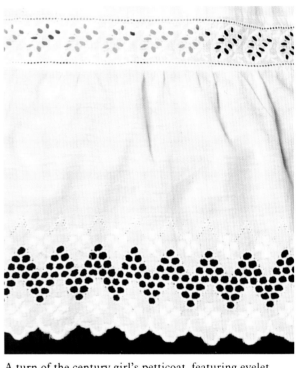

A turn of the century girl's petticoat, featuring eyelet trim. *Courtesy of Persona Vintage Clothing.* $30—$40.

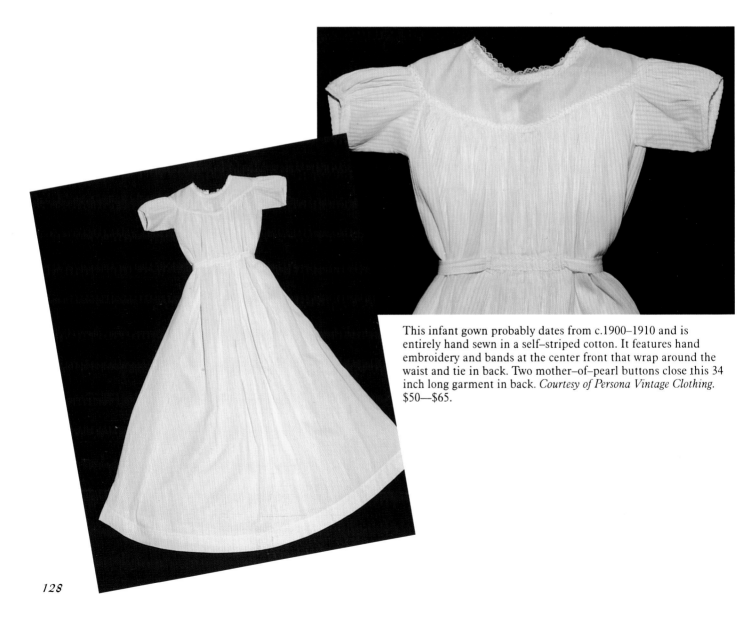

This infant gown probably dates from c.1900–1910 and is entirely hand sewn in a self–striped cotton. It features hand embroidery and bands at the center front that wrap around the waist and tie in back. Two mother–of–pearl buttons close this 34 inch long garment in back. *Courtesy of Persona Vintage Clothing.* $50—$65.

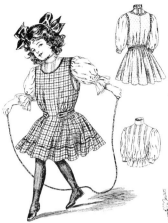

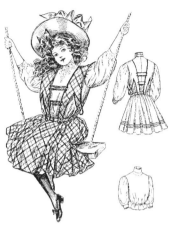

Two girls dresses, from the pages of a 1908 *McCall's*. The girl on the swing wears a two–piece dress consisting of a white blouse worn under a plaid dress or "guimpe." It was described as suitable for a six to twelve year old, and the pattern sold for 15¢. "A dainty little frock of white lawn with pale–blue stripe," was how the editors described the dress of the girl skipping rope. Suitable for a young miss of thirteen to seventeen years of age, the dress could be worn plain, or the ruffled petals on the skirt and sleeves (which were attached to each other and were a separate article of dress) could be added.

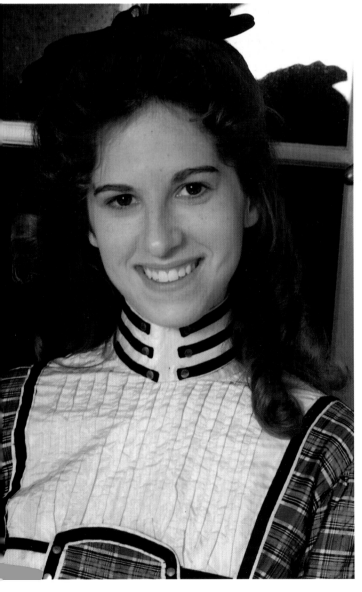

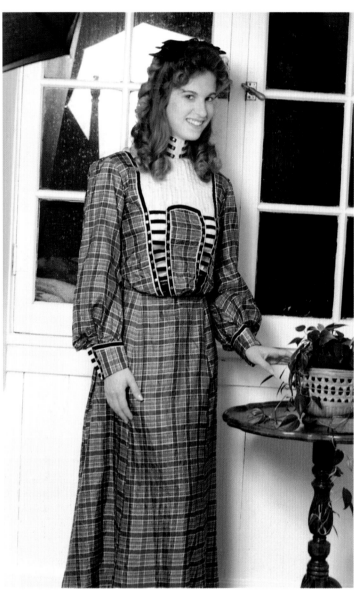

This young misses' blue silk plaid dress, c.1900–05, features a tucked white yolk. The collar, cuffs, and bodice front are trimmed with bands of black velveteen ribbon. The dress fastens with snaps down the back. *Courtesy of Vintage Silhouettes.* $150—$250.

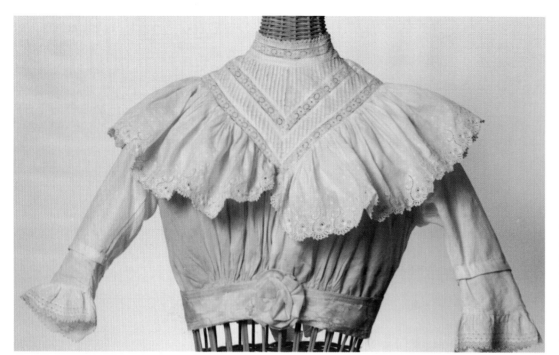

This girl's cotton bodice, c.1900–1905, features a V-shaped yolk of tucking and lace insertion, ending with a ruffle of eyelet. The bodice is slightly pigeon-fronted, and buttons down the back. *Courtesy of Pam Coghlan.* $65—$75.

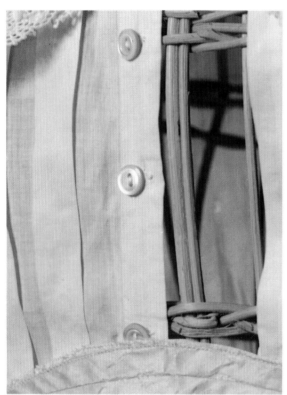

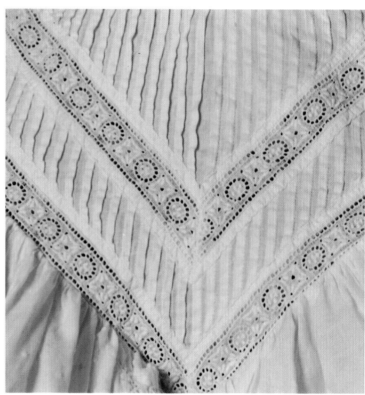

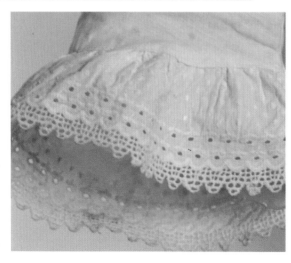

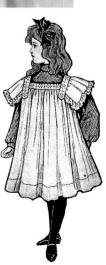

A "dainty apron" or smock for a girl one to five years old, from 1904.

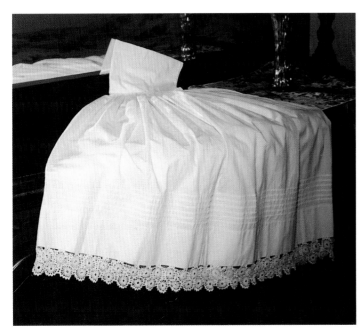

A cotton baby's slip, c.1900—1909. Slips like these were intended to be worn under christening and "long" gowns; the band was worn over the chest. This slip features hand crochet at the hem. There are no buttons or hooks and eyes; the slip would have been closed with pins. *Courtesy of Amazing Lace.* $50—$95.

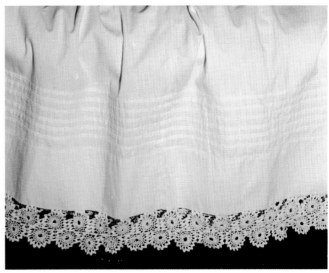

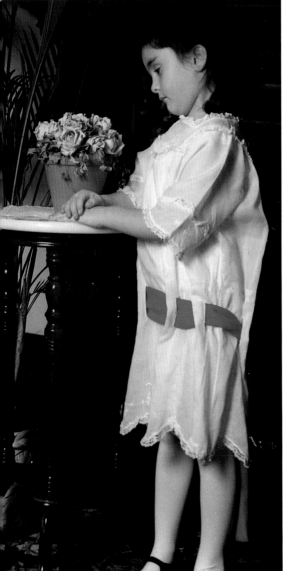

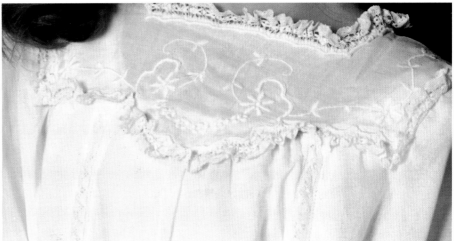

This c.1905–1909 toddler's middy dress features a squared neckline and a yolk featuring whitework. The short sleeves are also embellished with whitework. The dress closes with two 1/8 inch buttons in back. *Courtesy of The Very Little Theatre.* $25—$40.

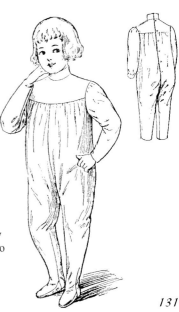

"As cold weather approaches," *McCall's* cautioned in 1908, "mothers are on alert for garments which will keep the little ones comfortable day and night." This garment was said to do the duty, made most appropriately in flannel. The pattern, for a child two to eight years, was offered for 10¢.

# The Birth of Modern Childhood

"It may be all right for small boys to go barefooted during the warmest weather, but even then care should be taken that they do not suffer from exposure mornings and evenings, and on wet, cold days. Girls should never be allowed to go barefooted, except as a childish luxury around the home, on warm days," one turn of the century mother's manual dictated. "It may not be so bad for little girls to go barefooted, but as a general practice, it can not be recommended as conductive either to health or modesty...Keep the children's feet well clad. Provide warm woolen stockings, and high shoes with thick soles...Children are frequently tortured most cruelly by narrow, ill–fitting, tight boots and hose...the little feet are misshapen while the bones are soft and easily compressed, causing suffering all through life...High shoes are better than low ones, as they protect the ankles from the cold."[1]

But it was not always so. Locke advocated barefootedness—even in damp weather; still, most children of the 18th century up through the 1880s wore rather high heeled (one or two inches) shoes. Often, in the 18th century and the early 1800s, fashionable children wore decorated or colorful shoes, and it wasn't until the 1820s that dark shoes were most popularly worn; in 1828, *The World Of Fashion* claimed that this was because they made the feet look smaller—though doubtless parents also found them more practical than colored or white shoes. Nonetheless, until the mid–1880s, white stockings (not black ones) were most often worn, even with black and brown shoes. Like so many other fashion trends, this must originally have been a way of expressing wealth (because white soils so easily), until eventually white stockings just became the "right" thing to wear.

To solve the problem of easily soiled white stockings, gaiters were sometimes worn. Popular from the 1850s through the 1920s, gaiters were essentially cloth leg coverings that buttoned up the side—like the more familiar spats (which protected the tops of the shoes), but running up to the knee. Socks were originally only for babies, and older children didn't take advantage of these garter–less accessories until the 'teens.

"As soon as it begins to get about on its feet, let it have little shoes," *Cassell's Household Guide* advised. "Very small pieces of silk, merino or Llama will make a baby's quilted shoes. Many ladies make such shoes for fancy bazaars. When the child begins to walk, let it have easy black kid shoes with

A single boy's shoe, c.1900–1920s, accompanied by a handwritten note: "Either Thomas or George Miller's copper–toed shoe. By the way the toe turns up, it would seem to have belonged to Thomas ('Tommy')." *Courtesy of Antique Apparel.* Without note $10—$15; with note $25—$40.

straps."[2] But the wearing of anything other than boots was, by this time, not recommended, especially for girls. "Do not allow girls to wear Oxford[s]...in the street, as they need the support of a shoe around the ankles," *Ladies Home Journal* opined.[3] This lead to much vexation for the child who had to wear them. "The worst worry in going out was my boots," one writer remembered, "which came far about the ankle with endless buttons that needed a button hook to do them up."[4] Lace–up shoes weren't worn until the turn of the century, and even then were rarely seen. Still, Alice Roosevelt had even stronger complaints about the sort of footwear she was obliged to wear as a child. "I also had a battle over footwear," she said. "Whereas other children had nice slippers—at least part of the time anyway—I was forced, for 'orthopedic reasons,' they said, to wear ugly black boots *and* braces, which I used to take off and hit the other children with. The braces were certainly due to the aftereffects of polio, which they didn't know how to diagnose or to treat in those days."[5]

Fortunately for children, however, by the 'teens zippers—a new invention—began to appear on gaiters and shoes, making dressing a wee bit easier. Though zippers were used on a few women's skirts and blouses in the 1890s (with the slogan that they allowed women to dress themselves easily), it wasn't until the 1930s that zippers became a popular feature in clothing. But by the 1920s, a new trend in child rearing was developing; it was now thought that children ought to learn to be more self–reliant, and to dress themselves from an early age.

In the 1920s, Ellen Miller, who dedicated her career to the study of childhood, noted that small boys had on average "more than seventeen buttons" to fasten each morning, many of which they could not even reach because they were behind or under his arms. Miller pushed the idea that "the independence and mental growth of the child should be stimulated by providing him with clothing so designed that he can dress and undress himself."[6] Nonetheless, at their rather crude stage of development in the 1920s, zippers were still too bulky and unreliable to be used in children's clothes.

Still, children's clothes of the 20s were far less complex than they had been even a decade earlier. Girls wore smock and A–line dresses; and they actually started wearing the popular chemise–style flapper dress in the 'teens—several years earlier than their mothers did.

Boys wore relatively simple knickers or shorts and shirts. Occasionally, young boys even wore long trousers like their fathers. Once again, most children's fashions were exact copies of adult styles—but now even adult styles had become relatively simple, and this making of children into miniature adults was far less trying for children.

Also in the 1920s, baby's often wore distinctly un–baby–like fashions. For the first time, babies were not always in dresses; in fact, they were more likely to be seen in rompers—an innovation that began in the 'teens. One can only imagine what 18th century parents would have thought of this style, since it openly admitted that, indeed, babies do crawl around on all fours. Too, the difference between a male and female baby was usually more distinguished in the 20s; little boys were unlikely to be seen in dresses and ribbons.

There were also other innovations in children's clothes; for all children of the 1920s, for example, the likelihood of wearing home–made clothes had diminished considerably. Though some ready–to–wear fashions (like basic baby clothes, and most accessories) had been available since the 1840s, it wasn't until the 1920s that the fashion industry began to flesh out sizing standards, really beginning to compete with custom–made clothing.

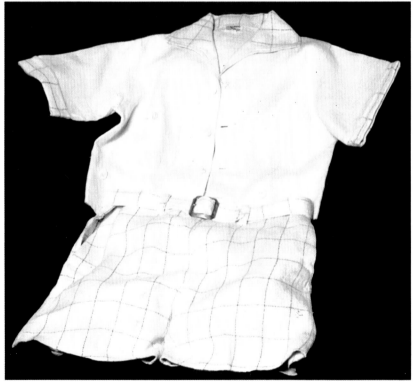

Blessings on these, little man,
Barefoot boy, with cheek of tan!...
From my heart I give thee joy—
For I was once a Barefoot Boy. *John Greenleaf Whittier, "The Barefoot Boy," 1856*

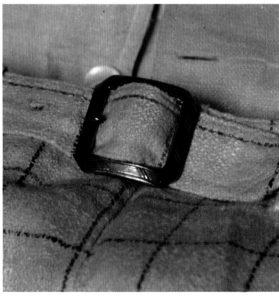

A c.1914–15 two–piece boy's linen suit featuring an "Oliver Twist" label. The shorts button onto the shirt, and the belt buckle features an Art Deco design. A 1915 Gimbel's Brothers catalog advertised many "Dickens suits" with similar style lines, and for boys two to five years old, they offered several "Oliver Twist" label suits. This exact suit was offered and dubbed "very neat and stylish [and] a fine value indeed" at 50¢. *Courtesy of Persona Vintage Clothing.* $45—$65.

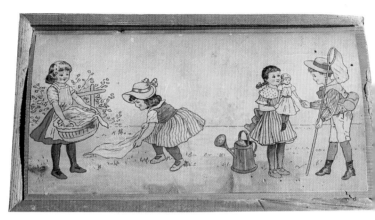

This turn-of-the-century wooden paint box measures 9.5 inches long by 5 inches wide. *Courtesy of Mother & Daughter Vintage.* $60—$95.

★ ★ ★

And so it would seem that in many ways, children's clothing has come full circle. In the 18th century, children dressed almost exactly like adults—just as they usually do today. Does this mean we expect more adult-like behavior out of our children, just as 18th century parents did? I wonder what collectors and historians one hundred years from now will think about our children and the way we dress them. Will they conclude we are too harried to fuss over ironing and the care of intricate clothing? Or will they favor the theory that we like the style and look of simplicity in our children's clothes? Will they think we have a strange love of advertising—so much so that we actually allow our children to be walking billboards? And will they, as author Estelle Worrell suggests, "notice the paradox that, after centuries of laundering diapers, we finally developed mechanical laundry methods—then began throwing the diapers away"?[7] We can only speculate...

### Endnotes:

[1] *Home & Health*, p.305
[2] *Cassell's Household Guide*, 1870
[3] *Ladies Home Journal*, Sept. 1902
[4] *Children's Costume in England*, p.204
[5] *Mrs. L.* p. 28–29
[6] *Zipper*, p.179
[7] *Children's Costume In America*, p.3

A c.1900–10 "Weaving and Paper Plaiting" kit in its original cardboard box. *Courtesy of Mother & Daughter Vintage.* $50—$75.

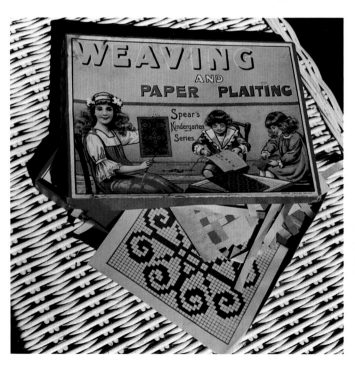

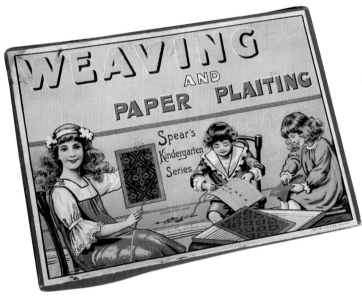

*The Christmas Santa Almost Missed*

In 1917, during World War One, the Council of National Defense decided an embargo of children's toys would save materials for the war effort.

Fortunately for American children, toy manufacturers, in shock and desperation, convinced the Council that toys like air rifles, cannons, and toy soldiers would only produce better future soldiers.

Impressed by the argument, the Council agreed, and Christmas of 1917 brought with it toys for both boys and girls.

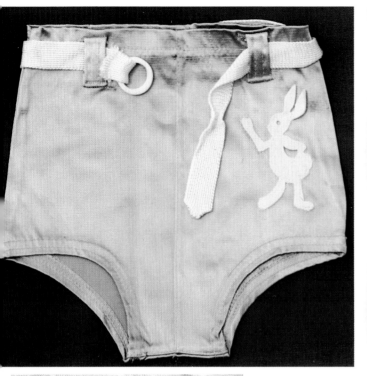

These blue satin boy's swimming trunks date to the late 1920s–30s. *Courtesy of Antique Apparel.* $15—$35.

The bathing suit is a 19th century invention. Previous to that time, men, women, and children either swam in the nude, in their undergarments, or (if on a unisex shore) in old clothes. "Some wear bloomers, buckled nattily about the waists, with cunning little blue–veined feet twinkling in the shallow water," one writer described the variety of styles on the beach, "others wrap themselves in crimson Turkish dressing gowns, and flounder through the water like long legged flamingoes; some wear old pantaloon and worn out jackets."[1]

It wasn't until the 1860s that adults began to regularly wear what could be called a bathing suit. For men, this was a one–piece sleeveless suit, covering the chest and reaching down to the thighs. For women, a more complex suit consisting of bloomers worn under a short dress was worn. Though children from fashionable families wore miniature versions of these suits, many children continued to swim in their underclothes or in the nude.

Until the 1920s, the wearing of a bathing suit when not actually swimming was rare. More often, while romping on the shoreline, adults and children wore their everyday attire. For children, this was frequently some form of the sailor suit, or simply a navy or white dress. Tiny shovels and pails were favorite accessories right from the start, but more often than not, children were made to wear hats, thick stockings (black was the favorite color), and slippers or shoes.

[1]. *Making Waves*, p.25

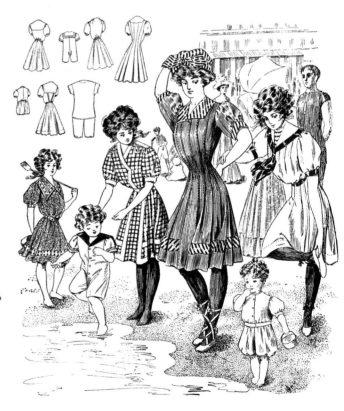

Bathing suits from a 1908 pattern book. Only the little boy (second to left) and smallest girl (second to right) are free from hampering skirts.

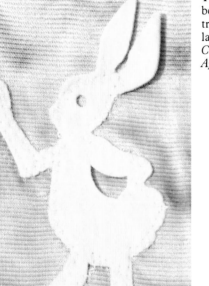

A cutting diagram and illustration for a ten year old girl's bathing costume, from a 1910 issue of *The Young Ladies' Journal.*

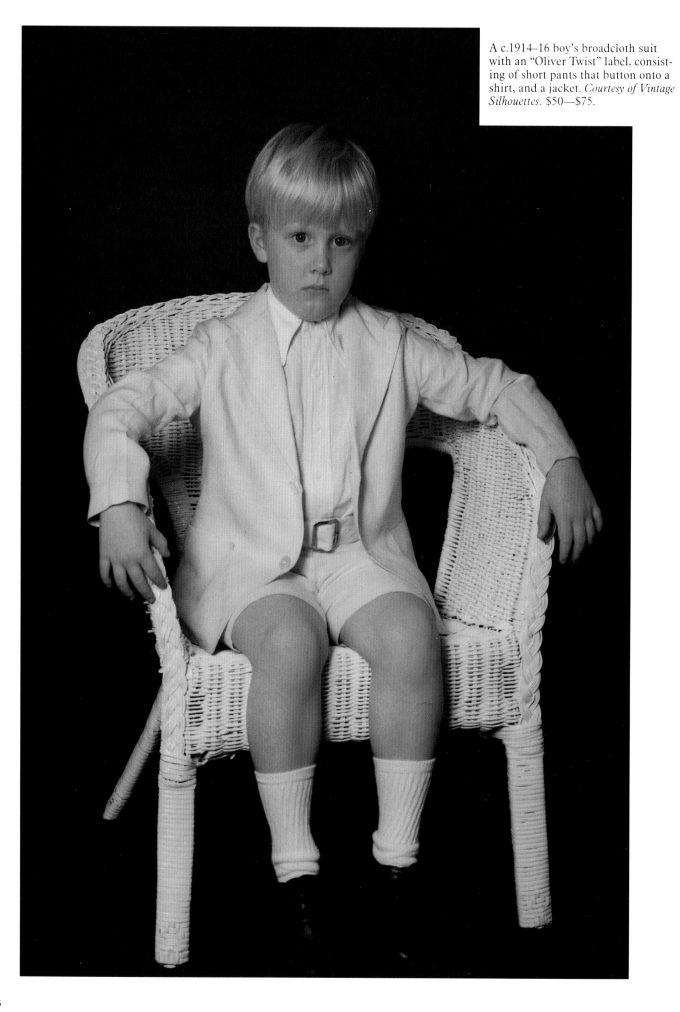

A c.1914–16 boy's broadcloth suit with an "Oliver Twist" label, consisting of short pants that button onto a shirt, and a jacket. *Courtesy of Vintage Silhouettes.* $50—$75.

## Busting Out

For the little boy, there is no more becoming a suit than that termed the 'Buster Brown,'" the editors of *The Delineator* opined in 1901.[1] Following closely the tradition of dressing children after storybook characters, the Buster Brown look first appeared when American Richard Foutcault's comic strip by the same name debuted in newspapers.

Featuring a toe–headed, mischievous boy reminiscent of Tom Sawyer, the comic strip found almost immediate success. By 1908, the Buster Brown suit—as seen in the comic strip—was common garb for boys under twelve years old: A tweed or striped suit with knee–length knickers and a double–breasted, belted jacket with a round neck, the outfit was completed with a stiff white Buster Brown collar worn with a floppy black bow tie and a straw hat.

[1]. *The Delineator*, Oct. 1905, p.31

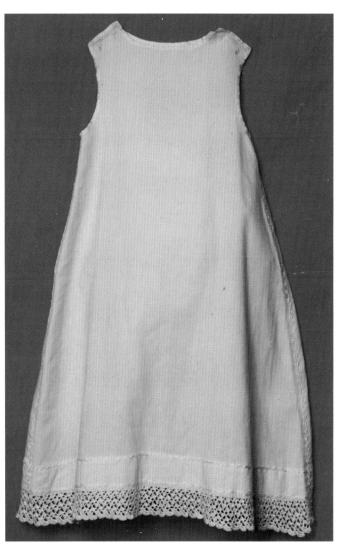

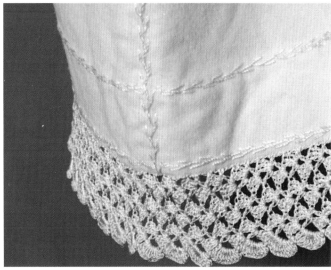

This baby's slip probably dates to the 'teens, but this basic style had been worn since the mid–19th century. Fashioned in wool, the slip's only trimming is hand embroidery and hand crochet. It is entirely hand sewn and the neck and sleeves are bound with ribbon. Two buttons at each shoulder are the only closures. *Courtesy Amazing Lace.* $65—$95.

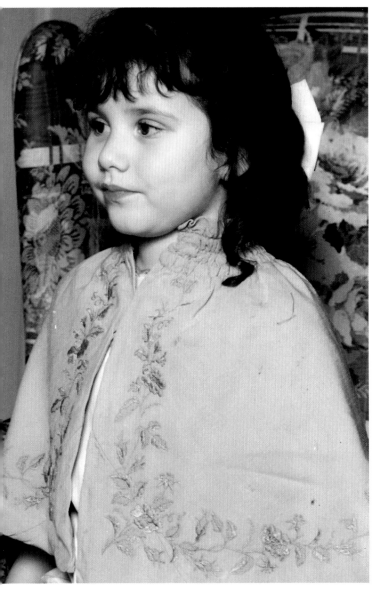

A c.late 1890s–1910s toddler's cape of flannel with a smocked yolk and tan embroidery. It is lined with a very practical grey flannel. *Courtesy of The Very Little Theatre.* $20—$35.

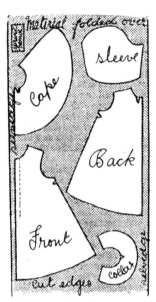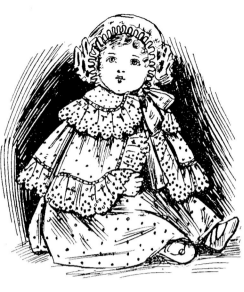

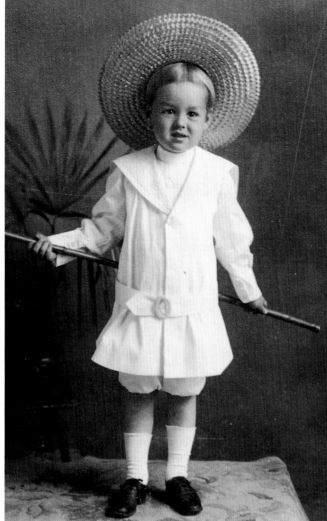

This cutting diagram and illustration are for a one year old baby's ensemble, and originally appeared in a 1911 fashion magazine.

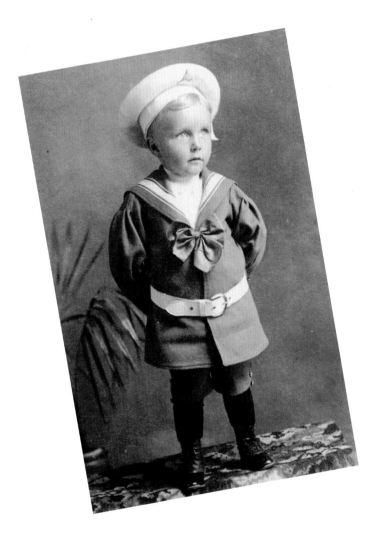

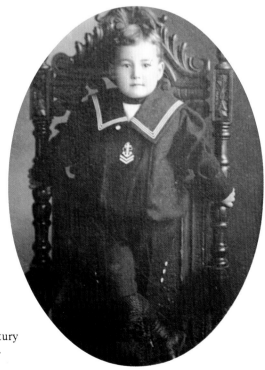

Three turn–of–the–century boys in sailor costumes.

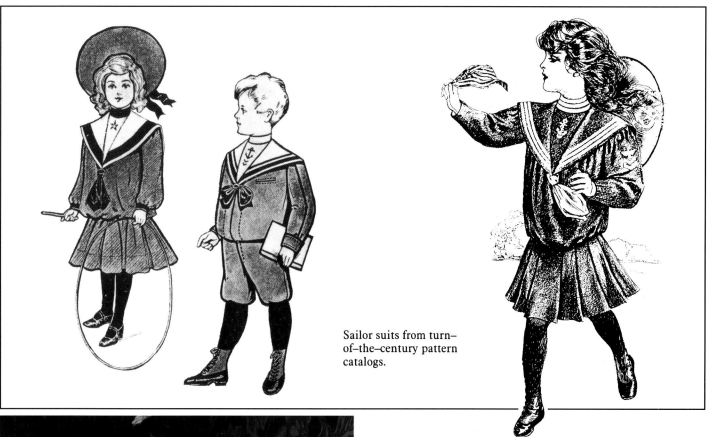

Sailor suits from turn–of–the–century pattern catalogs.

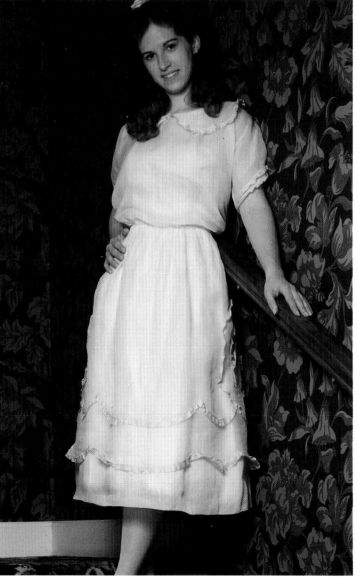

Like many dresses of the 'teens, this white organdy young misses' dress is lightly trimmed with ribbon. Near the hem, it features ovals of lace, each a rendering of a Japanese lady. *Courtesy of Vintage Silhouettes*. $95—$200.

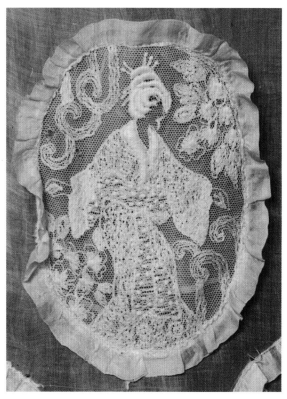

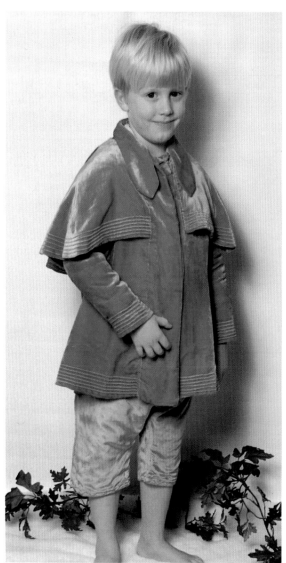

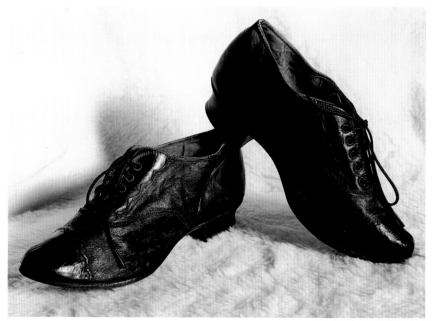

A pair of 'teens era black leather shoes, featuring a profusion of scallop accents. *Courtesy of Vintage Silhouettes.* $75—$150.

This 1913 fashion plate shows a typical girl's outfit of the era: a short, simple dress, with a "playtime" pinafore over it. $10—$20.

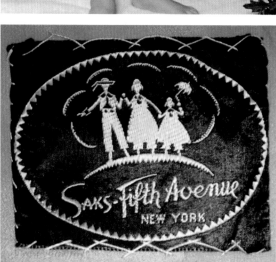

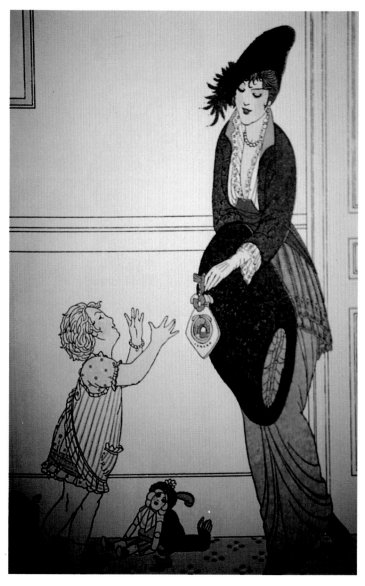

This boy's suit dates to c.1915, and is fashioned out of bright melon colored silk velvet. The flannel–lined short pants are trimmed only with V–stitching at the hem and scalloped stitching at waistband. The jacket features braid at the hem, sleeves, and cape collar, and fastens with hidden velvet–covered buttons in front. The jacket features a "Saks Fifth Avenue" label, and is lined in what appears to be rayon. Rayon was first used in 1912. *Courtesy of Vintage Silhouettes.* $100—$200.

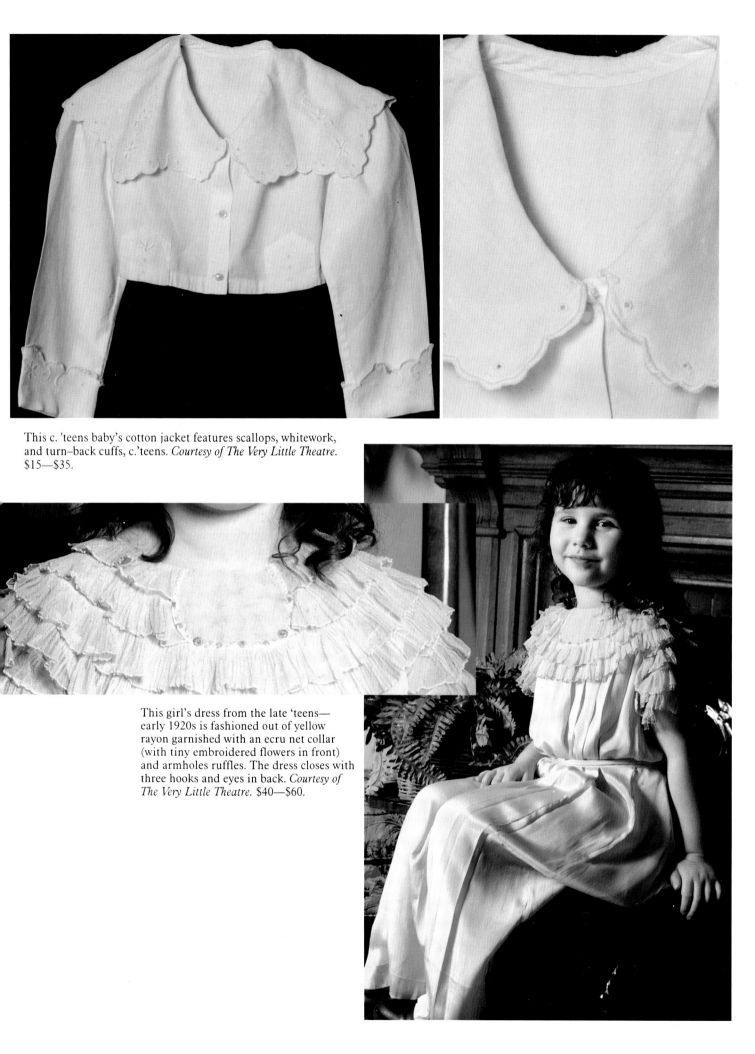

This c. 'teens baby's cotton jacket features scallops, whitework, and turn–back cuffs, c.'teens. *Courtesy of The Very Little Theatre.* $15—$35.

This girl's dress from the late 'teens—early 1920s is fashioned out of yellow rayon garnished with an ecru net collar (with tiny embroidered flowers in front) and armholes ruffles. The dress closes with three hooks and eyes in back. *Courtesy of The Very Little Theatre.* $40—$60.

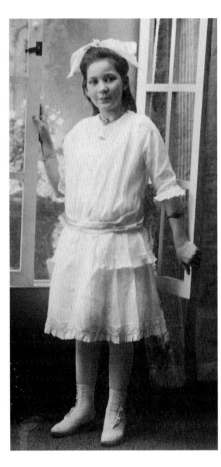

Dresses like these were at the height of fashion in the 'teens. The waistline is dropped (only older girls wore the slightly raised waistlines that their mothers wore), the skirt is flounced, and button boots are proudly displayed.

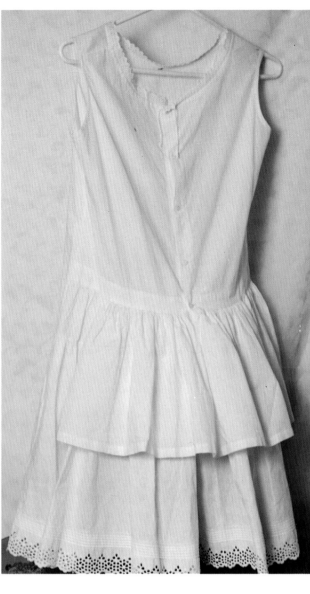

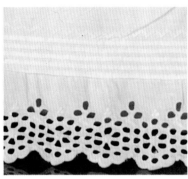

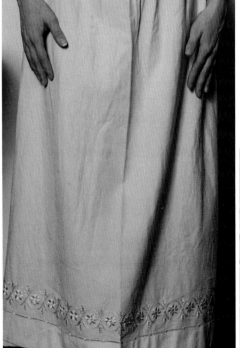

Two types of 'teens era girl's slips: The old–fashioned and the "new." The ecru petticoat is flannel, c.early 1900s–'teens, and is pleated into the waistband, which features button holes for buttoning onto the corset. The hem is embroidered with matching ecru thread. The white full slip from the 'teens is typical of what was worn under party dresses of the period, which tended to have fluffy skirts. The neckline is adjustable with a drawstring, and buttons run down the front. The waist is dropped and ends with a flounced skirt designed to hold out the outer skirt with as few petticoats as possible. *Flannel petticoat courtesy of The Very Little Theatre; full slip courtesy of Antique Apparel.* $25—$35 (ecru); $20—$35 (white).

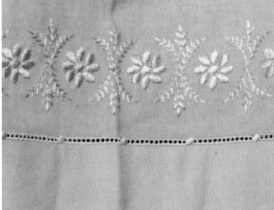

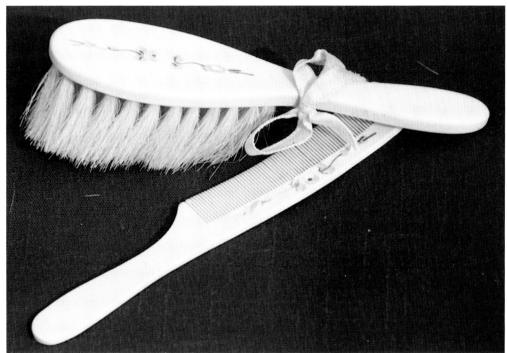

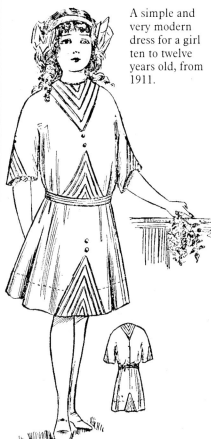

A simple and very modern dress for a girl ten to twelve years old, from 1911.

A dainty baby's brush and comb set, c.1909–1920s. Similar sets sold in department store catalogs of the mid–teens for 50¢. *Courtesy of Antique Apparel.* $20—$35.

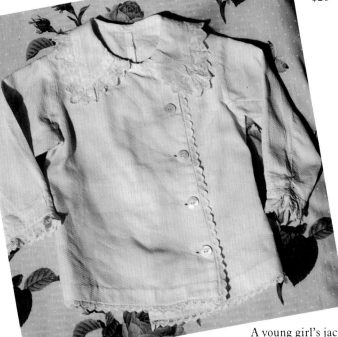

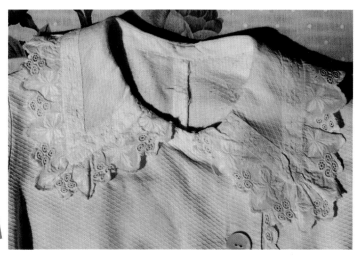

A young girl's jacket from the early 'teens. Trimmed with lace and fat mother of pearl buttons, it would have given its wearer the fashionable middy look. *Courtesy of Vintage Silhouettes.* $25—$35.

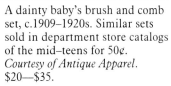

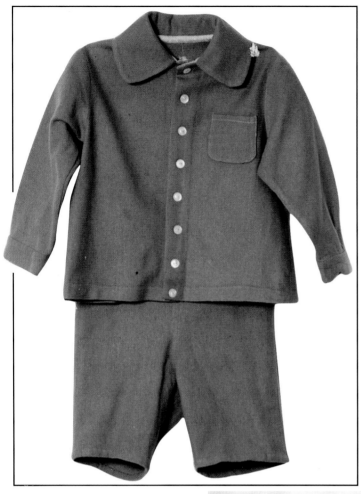

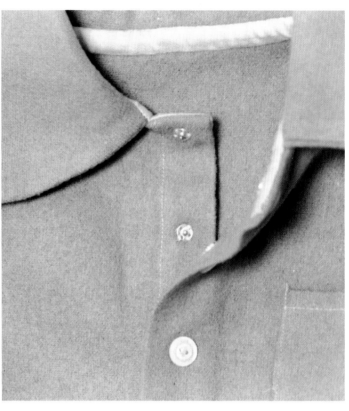

This boy's suit was very modern in its day. Clean and simple, it dates from the late 'teens, and like women's fashions of the period, it makes some use of snaps. Nonetheless, the trousers still feature buttonholes for buttoning onto a shirt. *Courtesy of Vintage Silhouettes.* $20—$35.

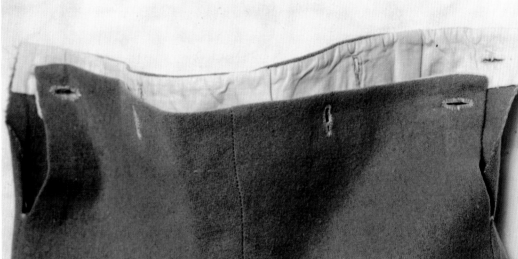

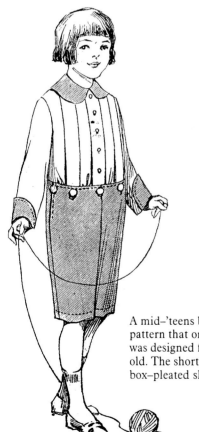

A mid–'teens boy's "Oliver Twist" suit pattern that originally sold for 15¢ and was designed for a boy four to ten years old. The short pants button onto the box–pleated shirt.

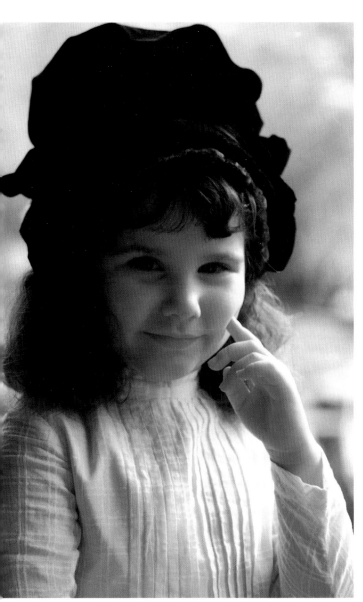

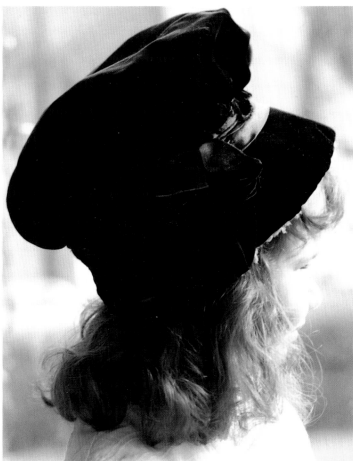

A c.1912–15 girl's black velvet tam–o–shanter hat with black ribbon trim. Sears sold a similar hat in 1914 for 98¢. *Courtesy of Vintage Silhouettes.* $65—$110.

Button–up leather boots similar to these were staple footwear for children from the 1860s through the 1920s. By the 1920s, most soles were glued on, not sewn on as in this example. The relatively modern opalescent buttons date this pair to the late 'teens—early 1920s. *Courtesy of The Very Little Theatre.* $40—$75.

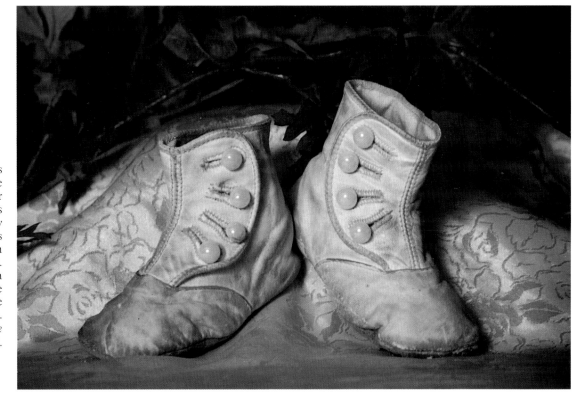

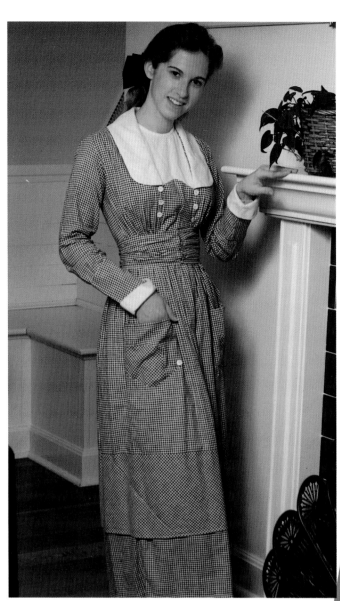

A classic young misses' dress, c.1915–16, in black and white check with white collar and cuffs. The wide, gathered, self–fabric belt closes with snaps in front, while the bodice closes not with the prominent front buttons, but with a side closure of snaps. *Courtesy of Vintage Silhouettes*. $100—$250.

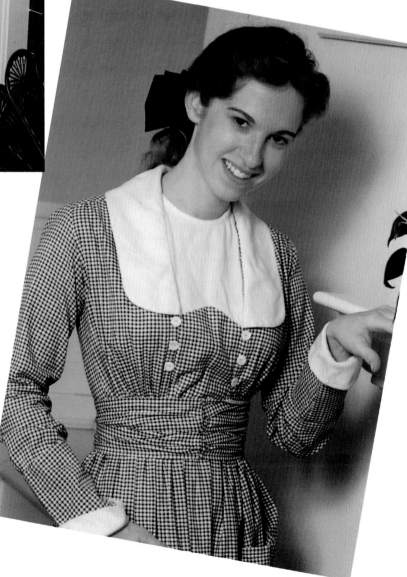

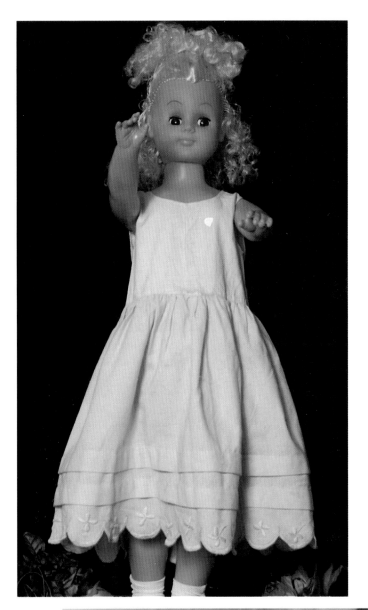

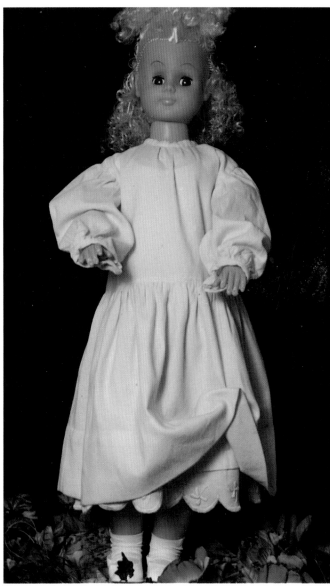

This flannel baby's dress, c.'teens—1920s, comes with a matching slip. *Courtesy of The Very Little Theatre*. $35—$65.

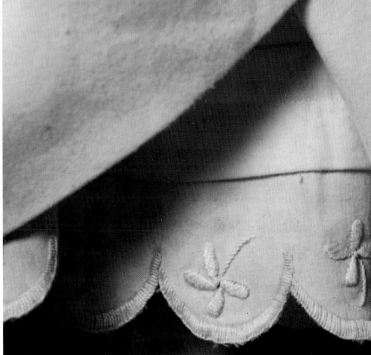

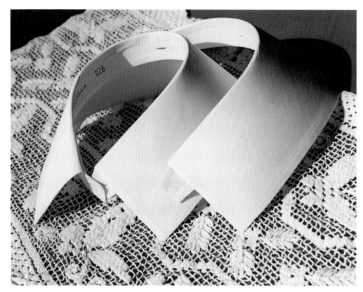

Boy's collars c.1900–1918; each is stamped on the inside: "Corliss...Tyke." *Courtesy of Vintage Silhouettes.* $10—$25 (set).

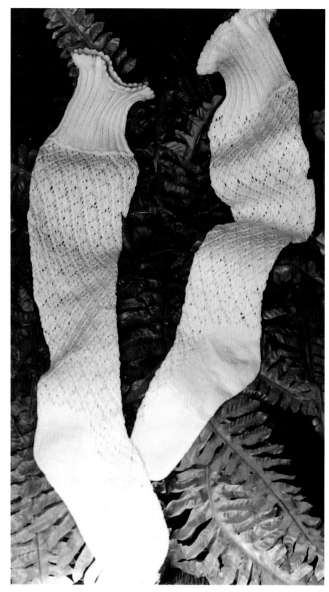

These girl's stockings from the early 20th century are of a heavy all–over open work design. *Courtesy of Antique Apparel.* $25—$45.

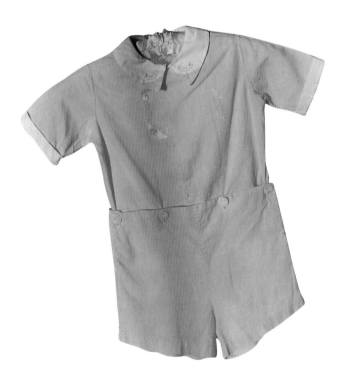

This little boy's peach–colored cotton suit with white collar, cuffs, buttons, and embroidered accents features a label reading: "Imported handwork, Handcraft." The unusual, geometric button closure dates to 1912–16. *Courtesy of Vintage Silhouettes.* $25—$35.

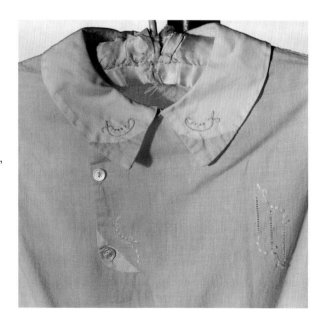

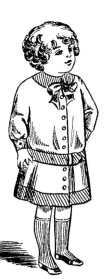

This outfit for a two to three year old boy was described in 1911 as a "useful little garment." Some of the buttons are functional and some are purely ornamental.

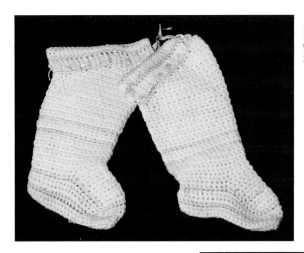

Hand made baby booties, c. 'teens. *Courtesy of Persona Vintage Clothing.* $10—$15.

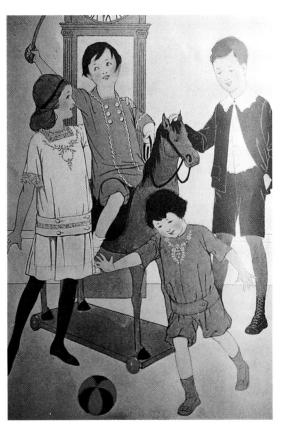

"Dainty Little Designs for Embroidering Children's School and Play Frocks," from a 1914 Home Pattern Co. catalog. The catalog stressed that "individuality may be given to the simplest of frocks by a touch of hand embroidery."

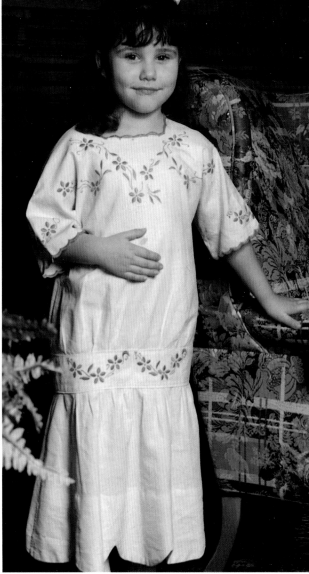

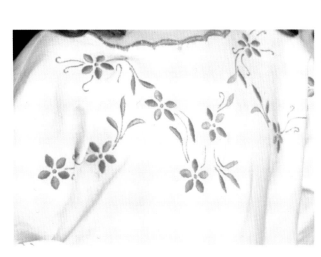

A typical 'teens era girl's cotton dress embellished with blue embroidery; the scalloped hem and sleeves are also typical of the era, as are the buttons that fasten all the way down the back. *Courtesy of The Very Little Theatre.* $25—$45.

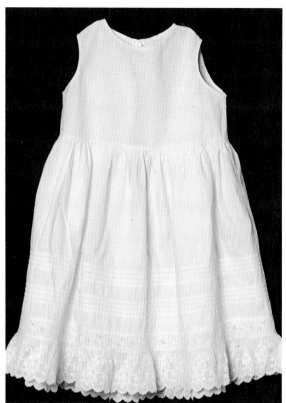

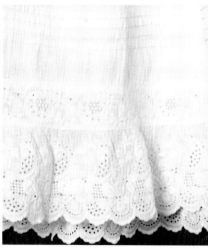

A c.1900–1915 baby's slip featuring a button back closure and a gathered skirt trimmed with tucks and eyelet. *Courtesy of The Very Little Theatre.* $15—$35.

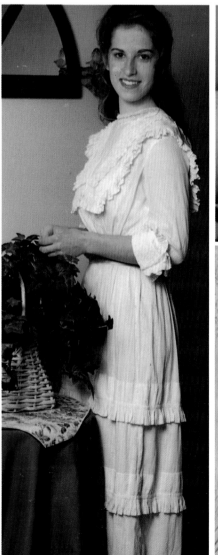

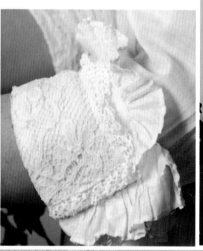
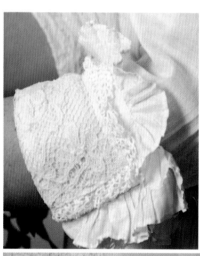

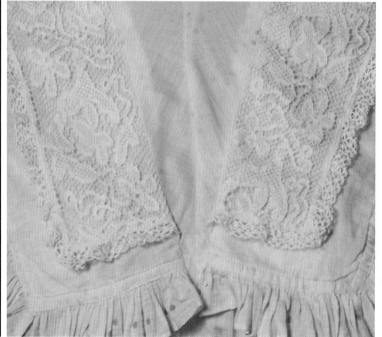

This cotton print girl's dress, c.1912–15, features a matching green satin ribbon belt. The dress closes in back with tiny crochet buttons. *Courtesy of The Very Little Theatre.* $75—$150.

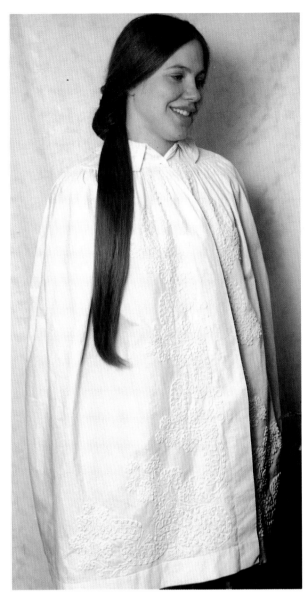

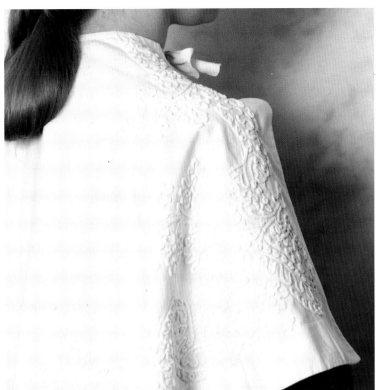

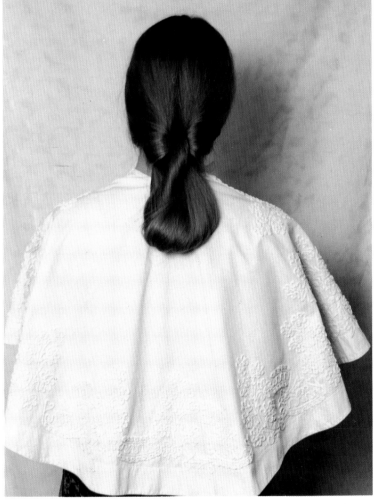

Sister's capes, c.1905–16. One cape reaches to the thighs, while the other is only elbow length—but both are trimmed beautifully with white braid. *Courtesy of Antique Apparel.* As a set $95—$125; individually $25—$45 (small), $35—$65 (large).

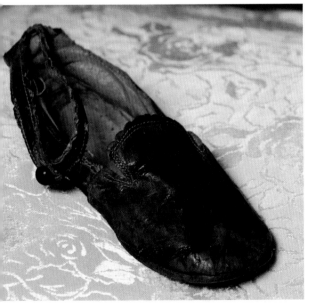

This shoe is a good example of how first impressions can be misleading. Although at first examination this child's shoe might seem to date to the early 1800s, upon a closer look it's clear that it's from the 20th century; the sole is not nailed in place, but glued. *Courtesy of Cat's Pajamas.* In current condition $5—$10; in very good condition $10—$25.

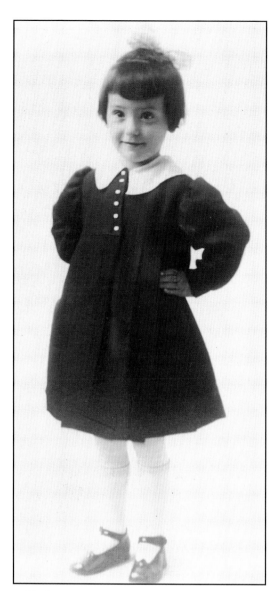

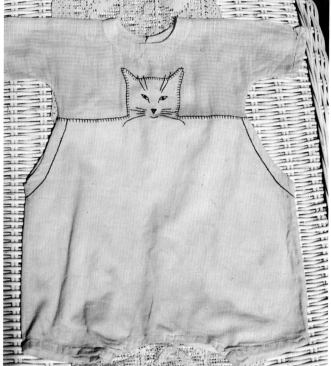

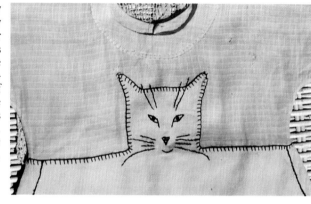

By the 1920s, baby rompers were firmly established as proper "everyday" wear. This cotton romper of the period is hand embroidered with the outline of a cat. It buttons up the back and features snaps for easy diaper access. *Courtesy of Persona Vintage Clothing.* $10—$25.

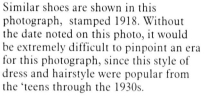

Similar shoes are shown in this photograph, stamped 1918. Without the date noted on this photo, it would be extremely difficult to pinpoint an era for this photograph, since this style of dress and hairstyle were popular from the 'teens through the 1930s.

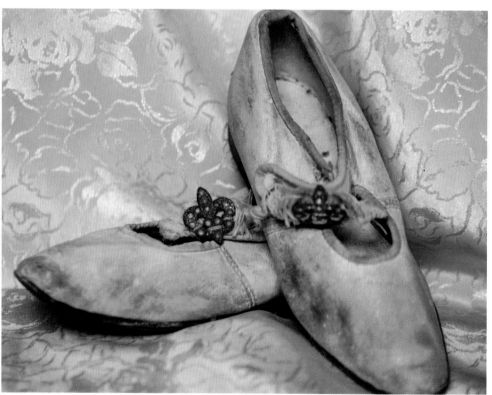

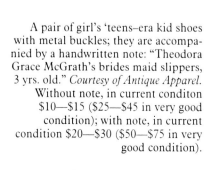

A pair of girl's 'teens–era kid shoes with metal buckles; they are accompanied by a handwritten note: "Theodora Grace McGrath's brides maid slippers, 3 yrs. old." *Courtesy of Antique Apparel.* Without note, in current conditon $10—$15 ($25—$45 in very good condition); with note, in current condition $20—$30 ($50—$75 in very good condition).

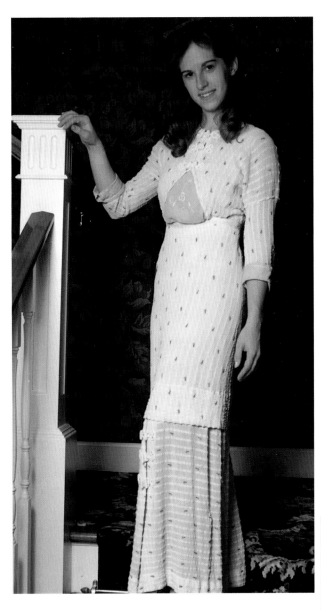

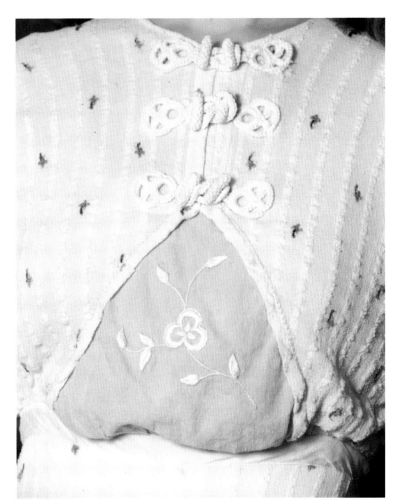

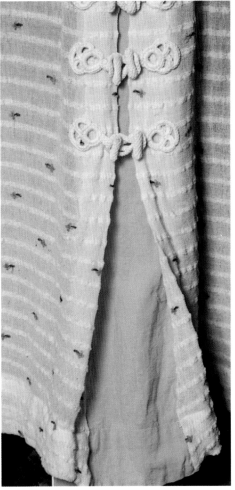

A young misses' 'teens era dress featuring lavender embroidered flowers. The frog closures are non–functioning; the dress closes with hooks and eyes up back. *Courtesy of Vintage Silhouettes.* $95—$200.

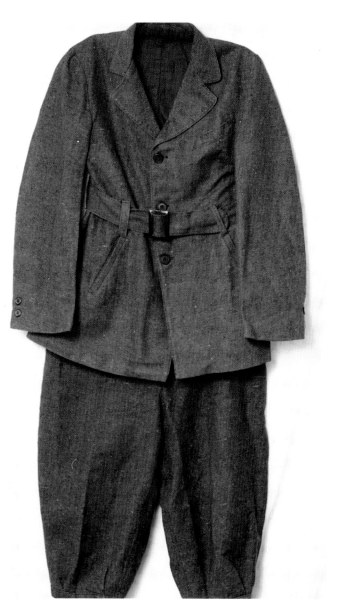

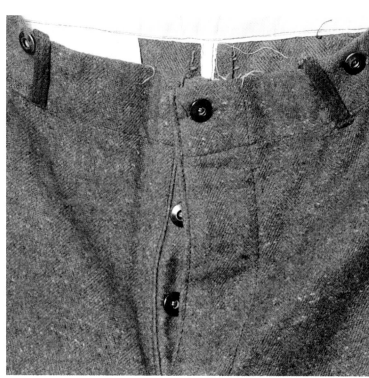

This boy's c.1910–1920s Norfolk suit is fashioned out of wool. *Courtesy of Antique Apparel.* $25—$40.

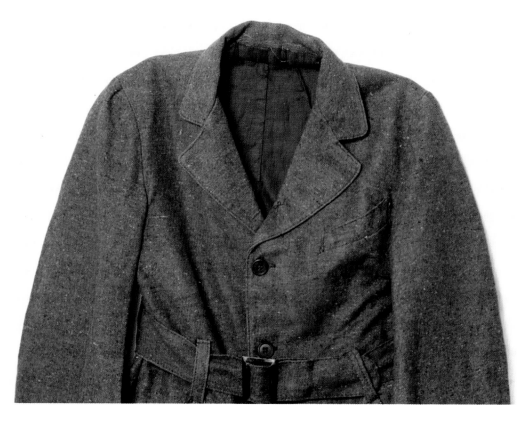

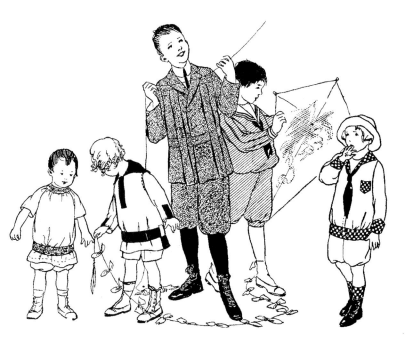

Boy's outfits, from a 1914 pattern catalog.

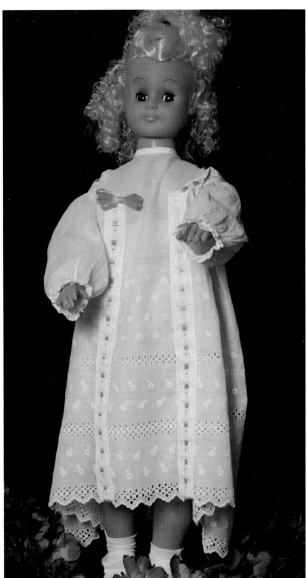

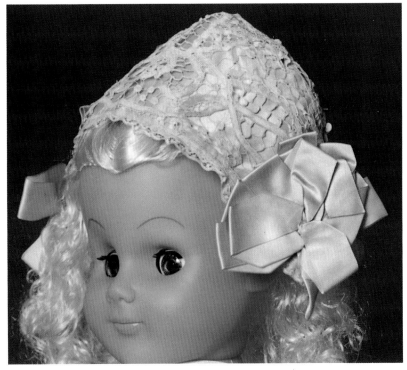

A 'teens era silver grey silk baby bonnet with an over–lay of lace. *Courtesy of Vintage Silhouettes.* $10—$25.

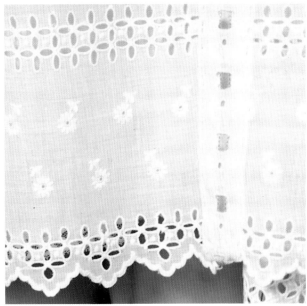

This c.1915–1920 cotton dress features with ribbon insertion and all–over whitework embroidery. In 1915, a similar dress sold in the Gimbel's department store catalog for $1. *Courtesy The Very Little Theatre.* $25—$45.

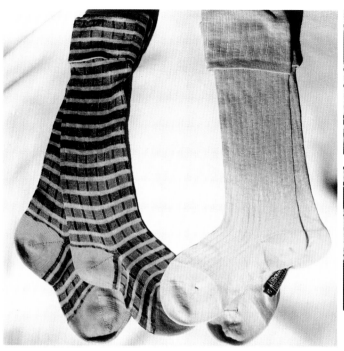

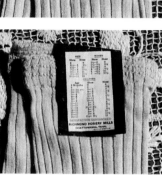

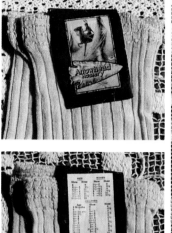

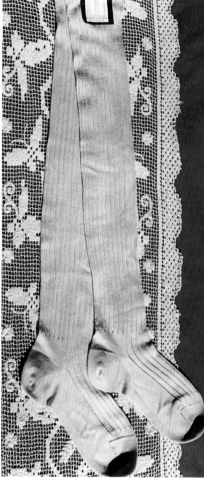

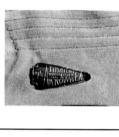

The cuffed, blue plaid stockings probably date to the 'teens. The plain ribbed stockings with their original "Arrowhead" labels still in tact date to c.1909–1920. *Courtesy of Vintage Silhouettes.* $15—$30 (plaid); $10—$25 (plain).

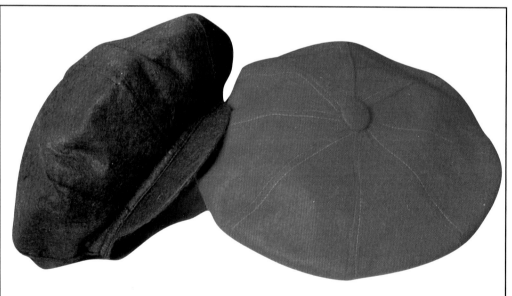

These boy's red wool hats, c.1910–1920, feature "Rob Roy" labels. *Courtesy of Vintage Silhouettes.* $20—$50 (each).

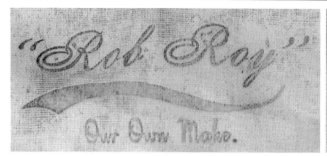

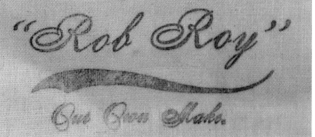

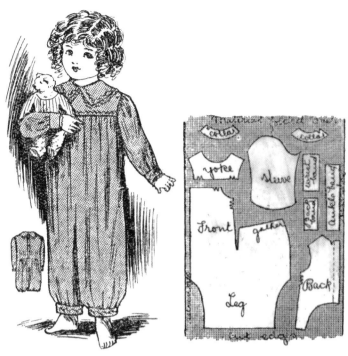

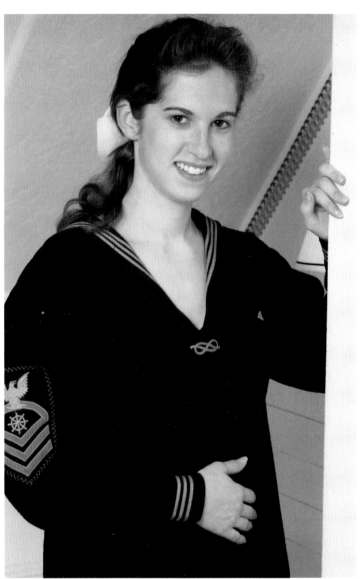

This child carries the newly–popular teddy bear and wears the newly–popular romper sleeper. The diagram and illustration were featured in the August 1911 *Young Ladies' Journal Fashion Supplement.*

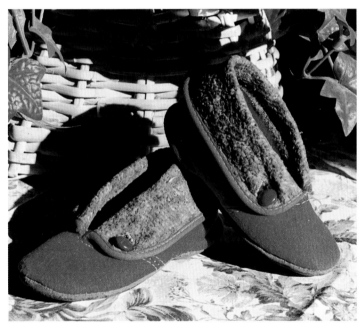

Red wool slippers, c.1910–1920. *Courtesy of Vintage Silhouettes.* $25—$85.

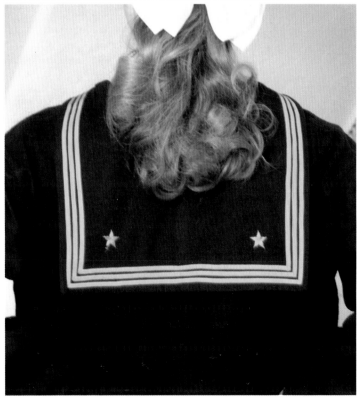

Military theme middy blouses, like this young misses' wool blouse with gold braid, appliquéd bands, and embroidery, were popular in the 'teens. *Courtesy of Vintage Silhouettes.* $25—$40.

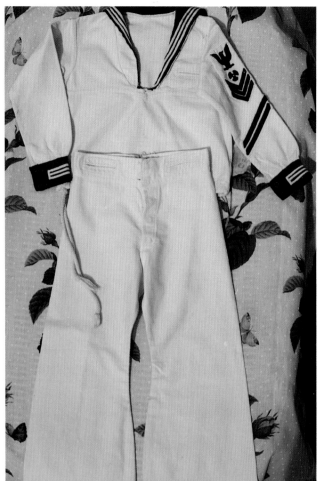

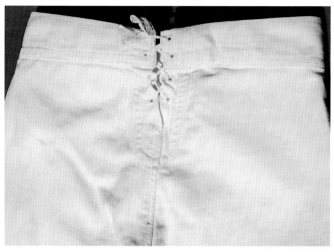

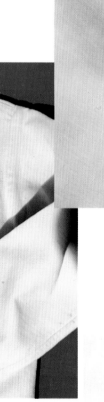

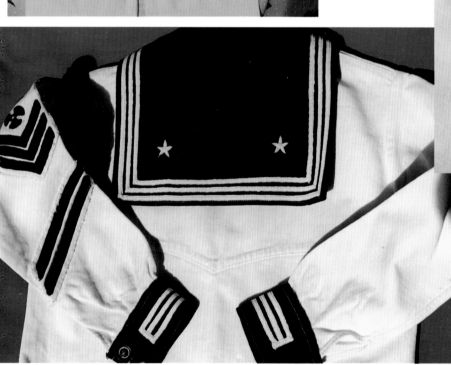

This boy's two–piece sailor suit is almost an exact replica of a man's genuine sailor suit. The suit is composed of heavy white cotton with navy blue wool trim. The bell bottom pants are laced in back, with welt pockets and a hidden button fly closure in front. Though suits like these were also popular during WWII, this suit probably dates to c.1900–15. *Courtesy of Vintage Silhouettes.* $35—$65.

A c.1915–1920s pair of girl's black leather shoes, with faux "alligator" like marks on their buckles. The soles are marked "Craddopck's Baby Lu." *Courtesy of Vintage Silhouettes.* $10—$25.

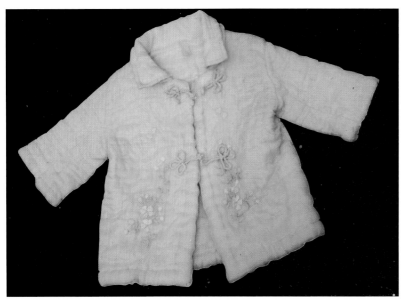

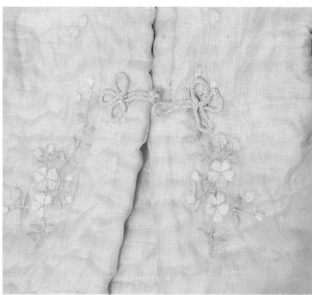

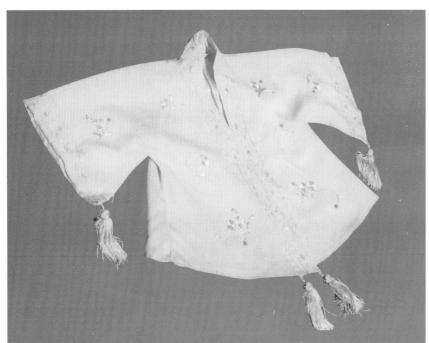

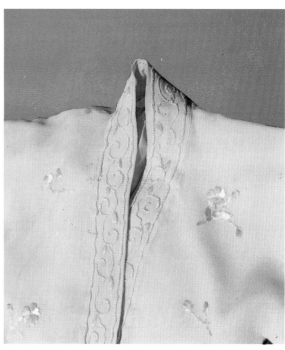

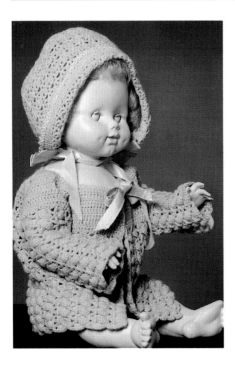

**Top left and right:** A c.1910—1920s baby's robe of hand quilted, hand embroidered silk. The frog closure is typical of this era. *Courtesy of Persona Vintage Clothing.* $20—$40.

**Center left and right:** The kimono was massively popular in the 'teens—1920s; men, women, and children all wore the kimono instead of a traditional robe or dressing gown. This fully lined baby's kimono is hand embroidered silk, and garnished with hand made tassels. *Courtesy of Amazing Lace.* $30—$50.

**Bottom left:** A typical hand made baby's sweater and cap, c. 1920s. *Courtesy of Persona Vintage Clothing.* $5—$15.

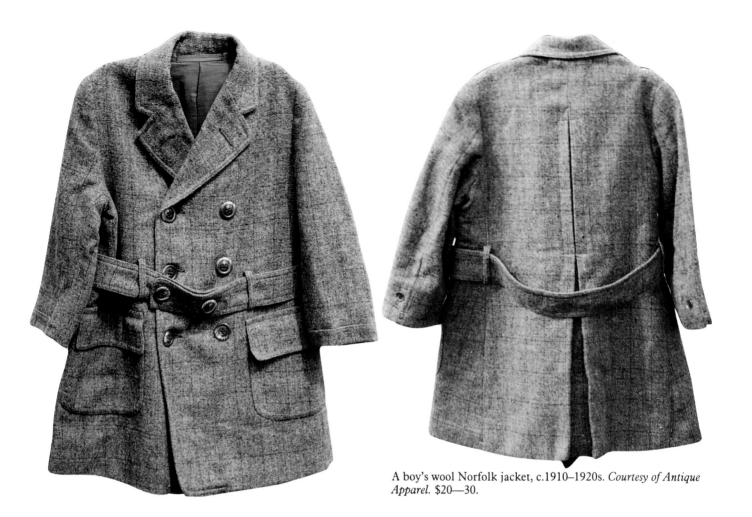

A boy's wool Norfolk jacket, c.1910–1920s. *Courtesy of Antique Apparel.* $20—30.

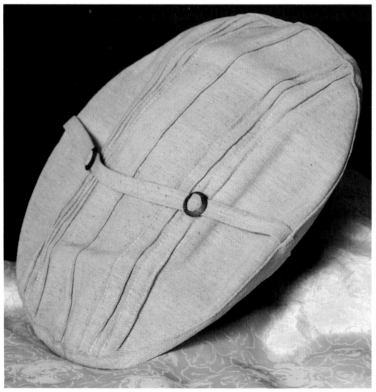

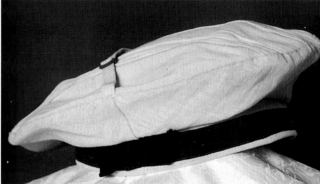

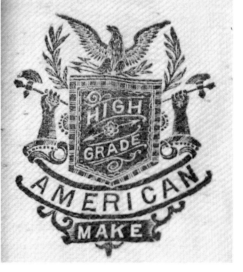

This c.1912–1920s boy's cap of ecru duck with a black ribbon trim is stamped on the inside of the crown: "High Grade American Make." *Courtesy of Vintage Silhouettes.* $20—$40.

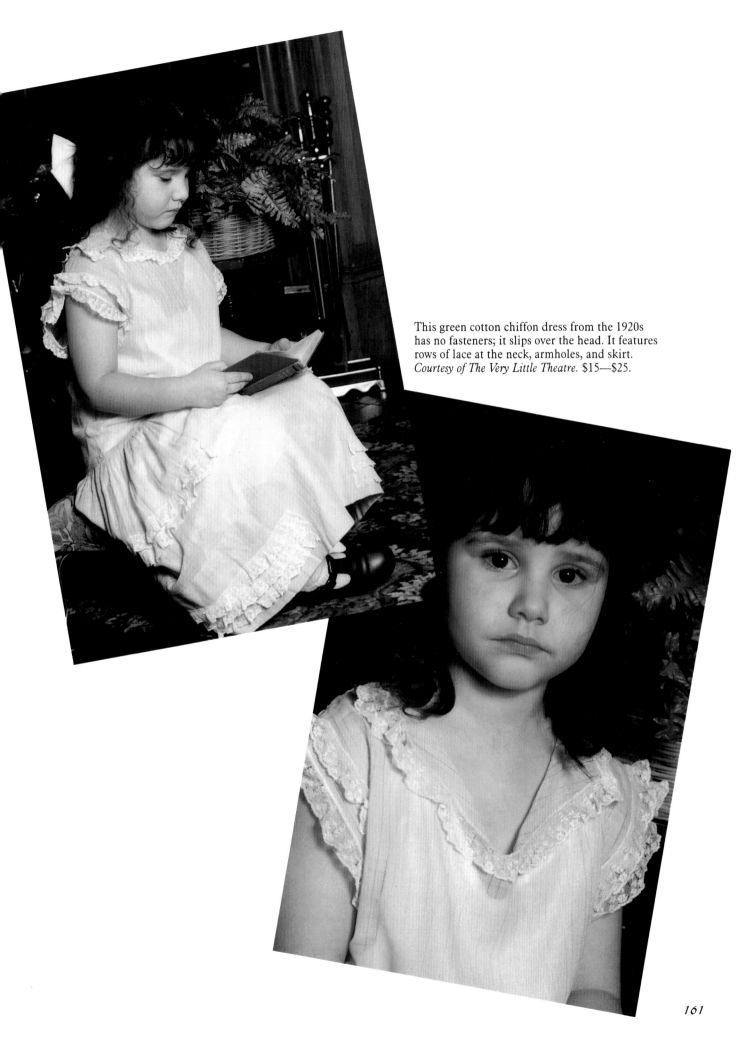

This green cotton chiffon dress from the 1920s has no fasteners; it slips over the head. It features rows of lace at the neck, armholes, and skirt. *Courtesy of The Very Little Theatre.* $15—$25.

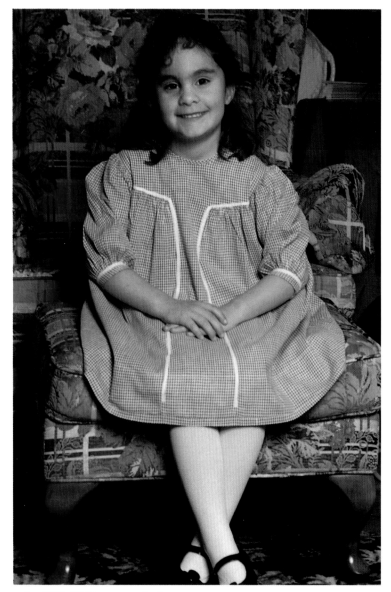

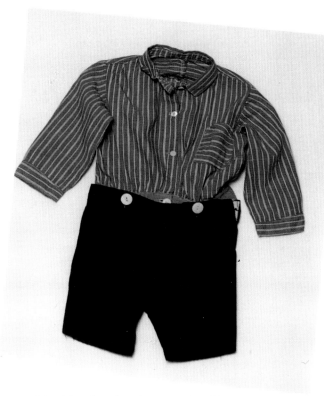

A boyish suit, c. late 'teens—1920s. The striped shirt buttons onto the shorts. *Courtesy of Cat's Pajamas.* $25—$45.

A c.1917–1920s cotton gingham dress, featuring a yolk that extends down the entire front of the garment. The dress' only trimming is simple white binding. *Courtesy of The Very Little Theatre.* $12—$24.

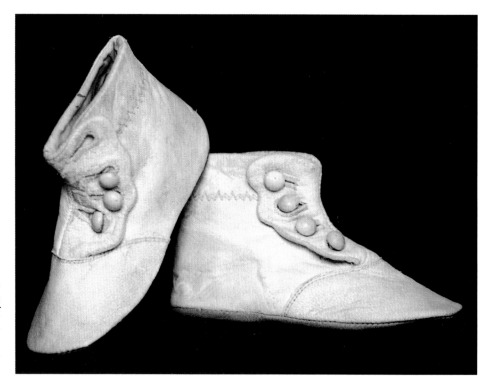

The zig-zag pattern sewn onto these kid button baby shoes is typical of the last few years of the 'teens and the 1920s. *Courtesy of Antique Apparel.* $10—$35.

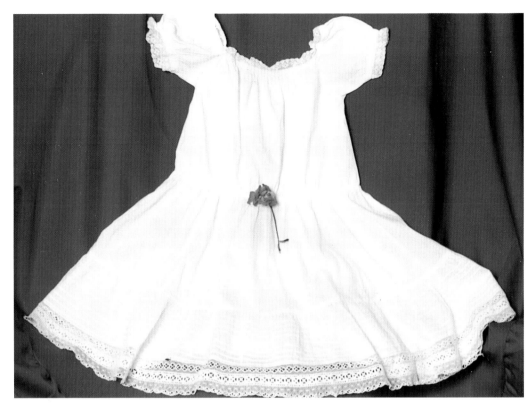

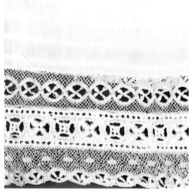

A c.1920s cotton dress with lace along neckline and sleeve ends. This style was popular from about 1915, but certain construction features (including the machine–worked buttonholes in back) are more typical of the 1920s. *Courtesy of The Very Little Theatre.* $10—$25.

A c.1920s girl's green chiffon dress with an attached slip. Delicate ribbon roses adorn one shoulder and the waistband. *Courtesy of The Very Little Theatre.* $35—$65.

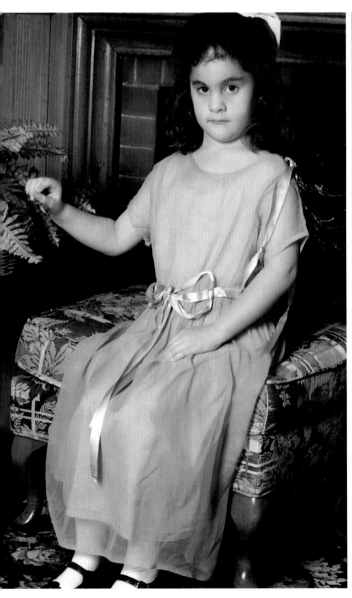

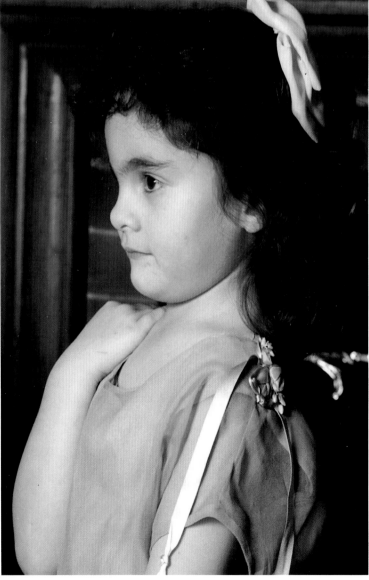

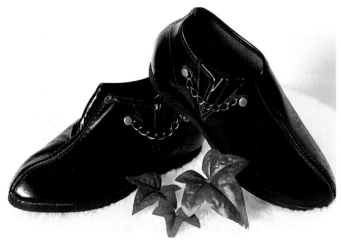

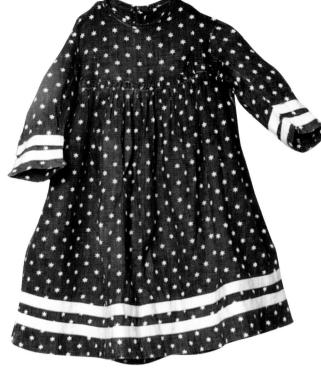

A pair of boy's c.1920s black leather shoes. There is a hidden panel of elastic where the metal chain hangs. *Courtesy of Mother & Daughter Vintage.* $15—$25.

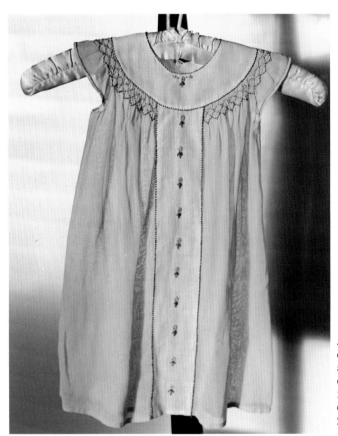

This c.1920s dress is fashioned out of star–patterned calico. The skirt of the dress has been gathered, the edge turned, and applied atop the yolk for a ruffle effect. The sleeves and hem are appliquéd with white bands, and the dress closes with buttons in back. *Courtesy of Pam Coghlan.* $75—$85.

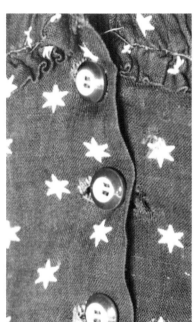

A c.1920s girl's sleeveless dress, featuring smocking and a center front panel with embroidered roses. The dress fastens with snaps in back. *Courtesy of Vintage Silhouettes.* $30—$50.

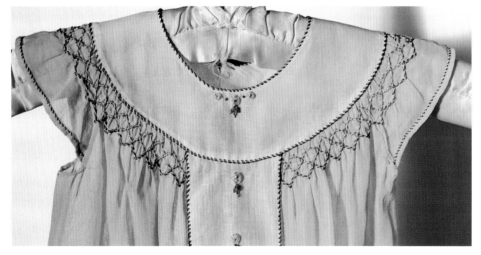

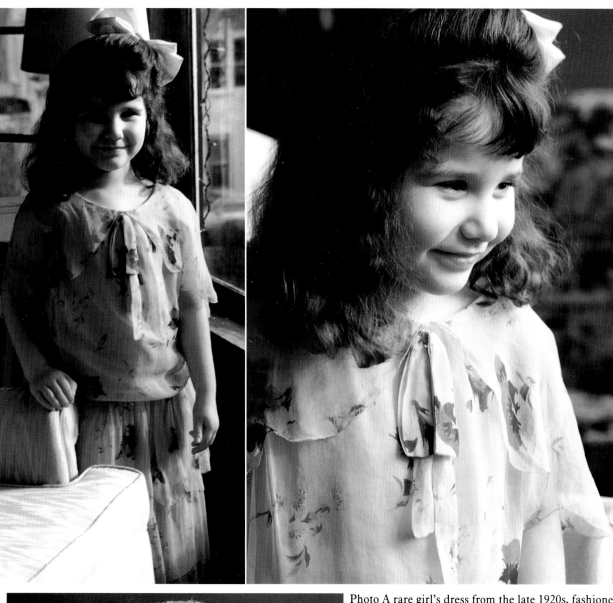

This c.1920s girl's dress of yellow print chiffon with a cape collar and a dropped and gathered flounced skirt is a miniature version of a women's dress of the period. *Courtesy of Vintage Silhouettes.* $44—$65.

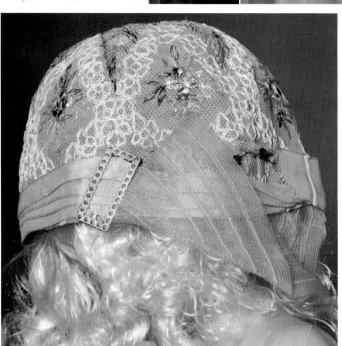

Like their mothers, girls of the 1920s wore cloches (or bob hats) over their bobbed hairdos. This pink cloche, fashioned out of overall embroidery and net, is trimmed fashionably with a silver buckle. *Courtesy of Vintage Silhouettes.* $95—$120.

Photo A rare girl's dress from the late 1920s, fashioned out of the cloth from a feed or flour sack. Though the tradition of creating clothing (especially children's clothing) out of feed and flour sacks dates back to the 18th century in America, feed and flour sack clothing was beginning to reach its peak of popularity by the late 1920s. The pinnacle of the trend was in the 1940s, and the fashion only waned out in the early 1960s. *Courtesy of Persona Vintage Clothing.* $75—$135.

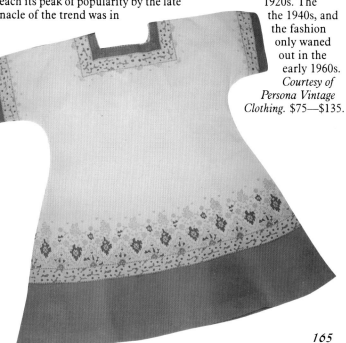

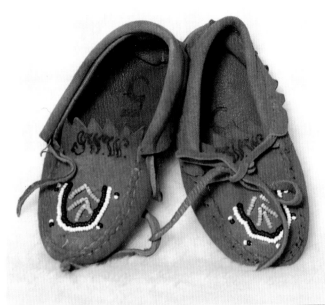

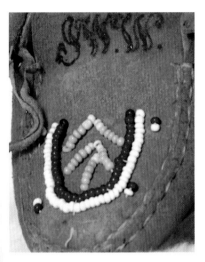

Leather moccasins made for the tourist market, c.'teens–1920s. *Courtesy of Vintage Silhouettes.* $30—$50.

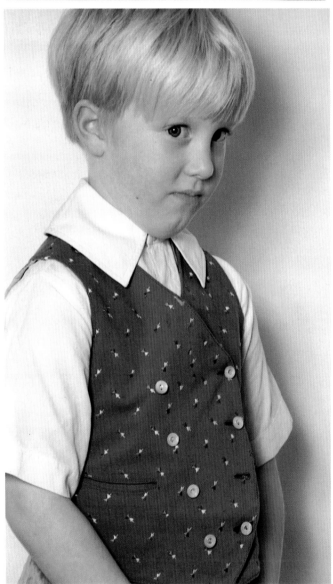

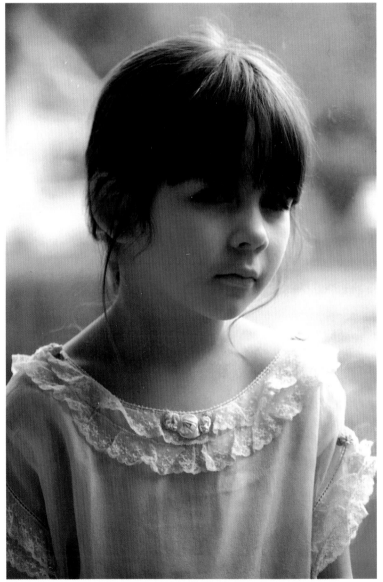

A c.1920s boy's vest of brown wool decorated with tiny embroidered motifs. At the back neck, a buttonhole is present for the buttoning on of a separate collar. *Courtesy of Cat's Pajamas.* $10—$20.

**Above and opposite page:** A silk chiffon girl's dress, c.1920s. Many children's clothes of the 1920s were trimmed with appliqués, embroidery, and—in the case of more dressy clothing—ribbon roses. *Courtesy of Persona Vintage Clothing.* $45—$65.

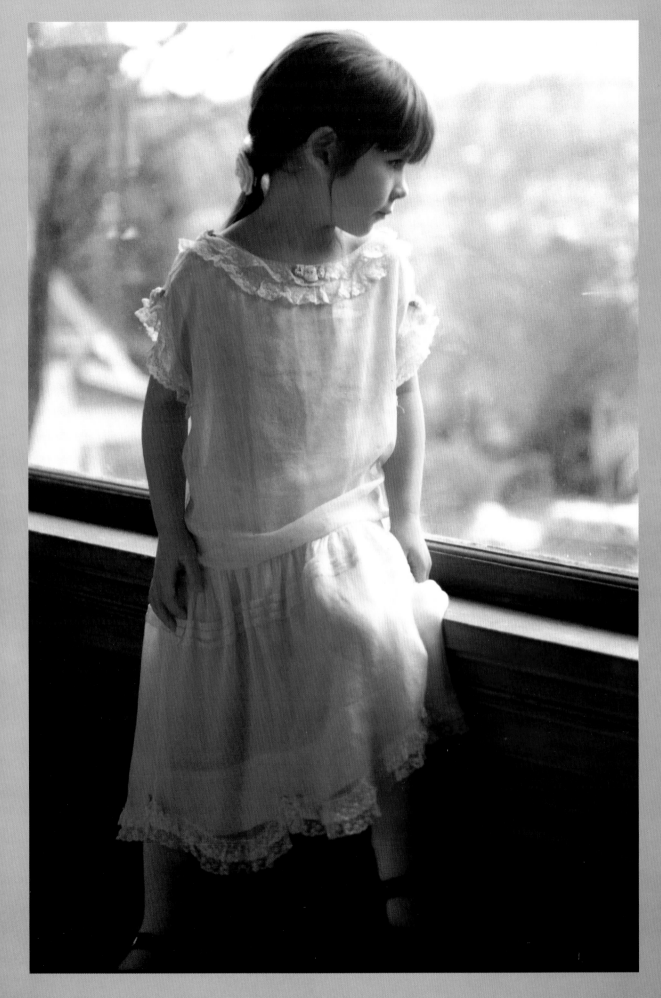

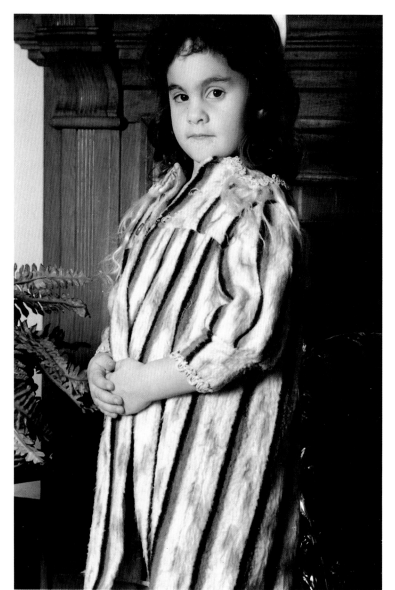

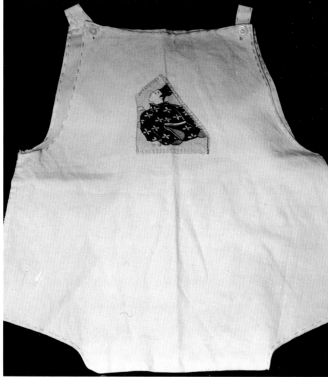

Bringing to mind Joseph's coat of many colors, this c.1920s girl's coat is fashioned out of a colorful wool blend lined in pink flannel. The sleeves and collar are trimmed with lace, and the collar is garnished with an unusual blonde trim that appears to be real human hair. *Courtesy of The Very Little Theatre.* $35—$65.

A baby romper from the late 'teens–1920s. It is fashioned of white cotton with gold embroidery and features an appliqué of a Japanese figure. *Courtesy of Antique Apparel.* $10—$35.

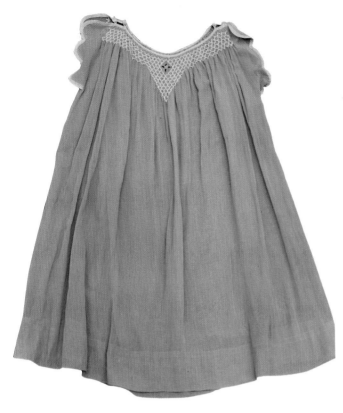

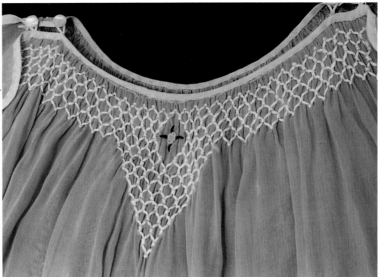

A c.1920s girl's green chiffon dress featuring smocking and embroidery. The scalloped sleeves and rounded neckline are bound with hand applied binding sewn with pink embroidery thread. Two buttons on each shoulder are the dress' only closures. *Courtesy of Vintage Silhouettes.* $25—$40.

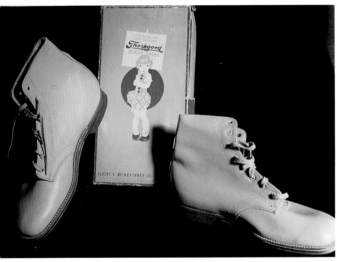

Dresses were simply made in the 1920s, unless their trimmings were extravagant, as these drawings from a 1925 issue of *The Fashion World* aptly illustrate.

These "Thorogood Health Shoes" in their original box date to the 1920s. The box reads "cute shoes for cute children, Albert H. Weinbrenner Co., Milwaukee." *Courtesy of Vintage Silhouettes.* With box $30—$45; without box $15—$20.

Black leather checked shoes, c.1920s. The pair on the left are girl's "Poll–Parrot" shoes, while the pair on the right are for boys. *Courtesy of Vintage Silhouettes.* $15—$30 (each pair).

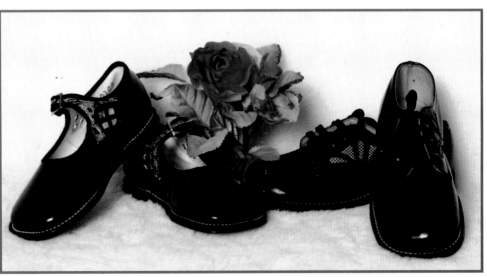

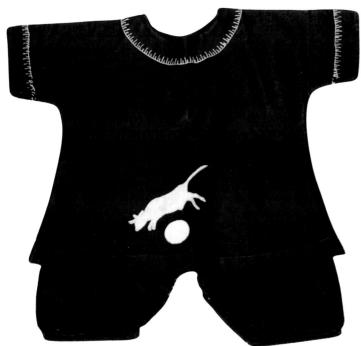

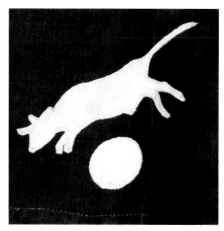

This child's playsuit from the late 'teens—early 1920s consists of plain black bloomers and a shift dress featuring embroidery along neckline and sleeve ends. What makes the outfit intriguing, however, is the appliqué on the shift: "The cow jumped over the moon." *Courtesy of The Very Little Theatre.* $10—$30.

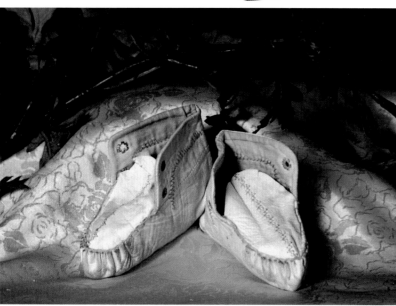

These c.1920s leather moccasins feature handworked eyelets and machine zig–zaged blue thread decoration, which match the blue cotton lining. *Courtesy of The Very Little Theatre.* $10—$30.

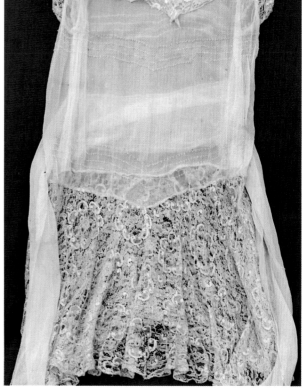

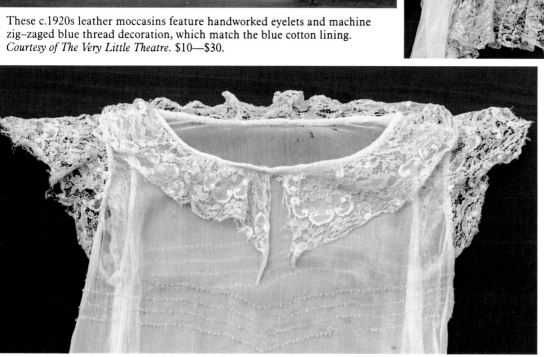

A girl's special occasion dress from the 1920s. The sheer pink chiffon bodice is trimmed with clear glass beads and features a collar and tiny cap sleeves of lace. The skirt is fashioned of the same lace and has an uneven hemline. *Courtesy of Antique Apparel.* $50—$70.

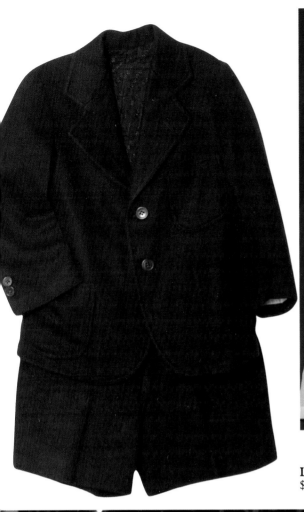

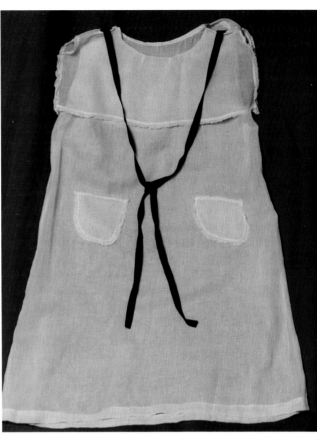

This girl's cotton dress, c.1920s, is accented simply with a white collar and patch pockets. The black satin ribbon falls down the front from the shoulders, where four hooks and eyes open and close the dress. *Courtesy of Persona Vintage Clothing.* $20—$30.

**Left:** A typical 1920s boy's wool suit. *Courtesy of Vintage Silhouettes.* $15—$35.

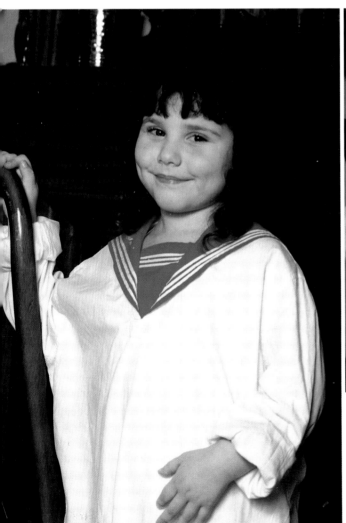

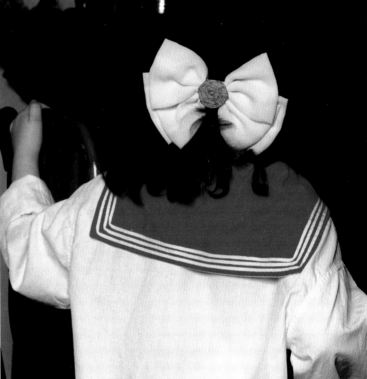

A girl's sailor shirt from the 1920s, featuring bright red accents. *Courtesy of The Very Little Theatre.* $15—$25.

*171*

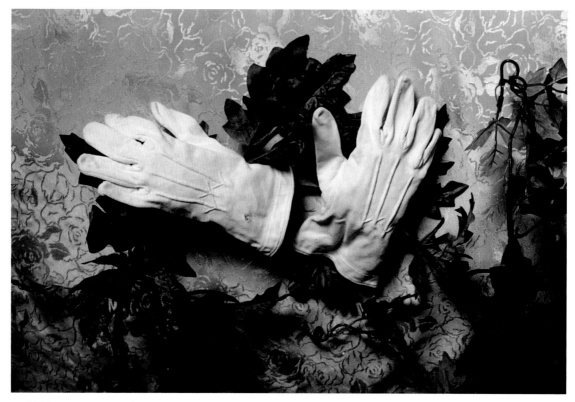

White cotton gloves from the 1920s, featuring a snap at each wrist. *Courtesy of Antique Apparel.* $10—$25.

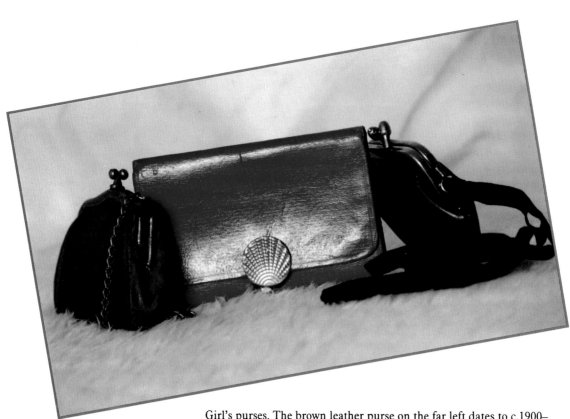

Girl's purses. The brown leather purse on the far left dates to c.1900–15, as does the deep red leather purse on the far right. The ribbon on the latter is of approximately the same date, but may have replaced the original metal chain. The bright red leather purse in center is c.1915–1923 and features a silver tone shell–like clasp. *Courtesy of Antique Apparel.* $20—$30 (left), $10—$25 (right), $20—$35 (center).

# Tips For Collectors

"One, two, button my shoe..."

There is something about those minuscule sleeves and tiny waistlines that makes antique and vintage children's clothing too darling not to take home. But whether you're a clothing collector, a doll or toy enthusiast, or an all–round childhood aficionado, there are certain basic things that you can do to help prolong the life and value of any and all children's clothes.

## Storage

Storing old clothing on a hanger is literally death by hanging. Old fabrics are always more fragile than they appear to be, and hanging puts excessive strain on the shoulder and waistline of antique and vintage garments. Instead, clothing should be stored flat in a cardboard box, trunk, or drawer. Protect the clothes from the acids in wood and cardboard that cause yellow spots by lining the storage area with an old white sheet or unbleached muslin.

With the heaviest items on the bottom, place the clothes in your storage area, being careful to put several layers of acid–free tissue between each garment. Acid–free tissue may be purchased from most art supply stores, and will prevent the yellow stains that regular tissue paper will eventually leave on fabrics. Acid–free tissue should also be used to stuff sleeves, pant legs, and any folds necessary to store the garment flat. This will prevent permanent crease lines. The tissue should be replaced about once a year.

Garments that are silk require a little different care. Folds should be avoided in storing silks, and instead of tissue paper, unbleached muslin should be used for stuffing or protecting the garment from the clothes above or beneath it. Many antique silks were weighted with chemicals when originally made, to make them seem heavier and more expensive than they were. This, combined with the fact that silk is the most delicate of all fabrics, means that many silk garments you come across may be shattered, or have large areas of tiny rips. Proper storage will help prevent shattering, but once shattering occurs, it is irreversible. To see if a garment is nearing this shattering stage, hold one layer of it up to the light. If you see what looks like tiny pinpricks or thinning, the garment is in a fragile state and will shatter shortly. To help prevent shattering, or to stabilize a garment that is already shattered, gently sew (with long basting stitches) a backing to the fabric; modern–day *coup de ville* is a good choice.

## Cleaning

Because old textiles are so fragile, cleaning should be avoided whenever possible. In fact, it is wise not to clean garments in your collection unless they are noticeable dirty.

Vacuuming is often the best way to clean old garments. This is done with a hand held vac whose head has been covered with cheesecloth.

Only cottons should be washed, and then only by hand using a very mild soap. A little Orvus (sometimes sold under the brand name "Quilt Care" in sewing shops) or Neutrogena face soap (which is what many museums, including The Smithsonian, use) in some lukewarm water, with a plain white pillowcase or sheet beneath the garment to help support it when it is taken out of the water, will do the trick.

Dry cleaning should be used only when all other means of cleaning fail; the chemicals used in the process dry out old fabrics.

## Display

Because of the size of children's clothes, they lend themselves well to home display. But care should be taken that they are not damaged in the process. Light of all kinds deteriorates fabrics; keep all garments away from direct sunlight or display lights. U.V. protected glass is available if you frame some items, and should effectively protect the garments from fading and deterioration.

Dust is also the enemy of fabric, as is moisture. The latter means that clothing should never be displayed or stored in the kitchen, bathroom, attic, or basement.

It is also a good idea to rotate your displays frequently. Remember that fabrics (unless they are entirely man–made) are literally dying from the moment they are made. This is why museums rarely have permanent costume displays, and keep their collection in storage throughout most of the year.

With this little bit of extra care, your collection of children's fashions can educate and bring "oohs" and "ahs" and "oh–how–cute"s to many generations to come.

"Buttons, a farthing a pair!
Come, who will buy them of me?
They're round and sound and pretty,
And fit for girls of the city.
Come, who will buy them of me?"

# Select Bibliography

**Books:**

Alcott, Louisa May. *Jack and Jill.* Little, Brown, and Co., Boston, 1869.

*Altman's Spring & Summer Fashions Catalog* [reprint]. Dover Publications, New York, 1995.

Ariès, Philippe, and George Duby. *History of Private Life, A.* Harvard University Press, Cambridge, Massachusettes, 1989.

*Art of Dressmaking, The.* Butterick Publishing Co., New York, 1927.

Black, Alexander. *Modern Daughters.* Charles Scribner's Sons, New York, 1899.

*Bloomingdale's Illustrated 1886 Catalog* [reprint]. Dover Publications, New York, 1988.

Blum, Stella (ed.). *Ackermann's Costume Plates: Women's Fashions in England, 1818–1828.* Dover Publications, New York, 1978.

——————(ed.). *Everyday Fashions of the Twenties as Pictured in Sears and Other Catalogs.* Dover Publications, New York, 1981.

——————(ed.). *Fashions and Costumes From Godey's Lady's Book.* Dover Publications, New York, 1985.

——————(ed.). *Victorian Fashions and Costumes from Harper's Bazar, 1867–1898.* Dover Publications, New York, 1974.

Bonebright, Sarah. *Reminiscences of Newcastle, Iowa.* Des Moines, 1921, Historical Department of Iowa.

Chopin, Kate. *The Awakening* [reprint]. Avon Books, New York, 1972.

Cunnington, C.W. and Phillis. *History of Underclothes, The* [reprint]. Dover Publications, New York, 1992.

Cunnington, Phillis and Anne Buck. *Children's Costume in England.* Barnes & Noble, New York, 1965.

Dalrymple, Priscilla Harris. *American Victorian Costume in Early Photographs.* Dover Publications, New York, 1991.

Drake, Emma F. Angell, M.D. *What A Young Wife Ought To Know.* Vir Publishing Co., Philadelphia, 1908.

*Dressmaking, Up To Date.* Butterick Publishing Co., New York, 1905.

Ewing, Elizabeth. *History of Children's Costume.* Charles Scribner's Sons, New York, 1977.

*Franklin Simon Fashion Catalog for 1923* [reprint]. Dover Publications, New York, 1993.

Fraser, Antonia. *Weaker Vessel, The.* Random House, New York, 1984.

Friedel, Robert. *Zipper.* W.W. Norton & Co., New York, 1994.

Gattey, Charles Neilson. *The Bloomer Girls.* Coward–McCann, Inc., New York, 1967.

Gernsheim, Alison. *Victorian and Edwardian Fashion: A Photographic Survey.* Dover Publications, New York, 1981.

Green, Harvey. *Light of The Home, The.* Patheon Books, New York, 1983.

Hall, Lee. *Common Threads.* Little, Brown, & Co., Boston, 1992.

Harris, Kristina. *59 Authentic Turn-of-the-Century Fashion Patterns.* Dover Publications, New York, 1994.

——————(ed.). *Home Pattern Company 1914 Fashion Catalog, The* [reprint]. Dover Publications, New York, 1995.

——————. *Victorian & Edwardian Fashions For Women: 1840–1919.* Schiffer Publishing, Atglen, Pennsylvania, 1995.

——————. *Vintage Fashions For Women: 1920s—1940s.* Schiffer Publishing, Atglen, Pennsylvania, 1996.

Hartley, Florence. *Ladies' Book of Etiquette, The* [reprint of 1860 edition]. Amazon Dry Goods, Davenport, IA, 1993

Heininger, Mary Lynn Stevens, Karin Calvert, Barbara Finkelstein, Kathy Vandell, Anne Scott MacLeod, and Harvey Green. *Century of Childhood, A.* Margaret Woodbury Strong Museum, Rochester, New York, 1984.

Holme, Bryan. *The Kate Greenway Book.* Viking Press, New York, 1976.

*Home and Health.* Pacific Press Publishing Co., Mountain View, CA, 1907.

Hunt, Una. *Una May.* Charles Scribner's Sons, New York, 1914.

Jarvis, Anthea and Patricia Raine. *Fancy Dress.* Shire Publications, London, 1984.

Kidwell, Claudia Brush and Valerie Steele. *Men & Women.* Smithsonian Institution Press, Washington DC, 1989.

Kybalová, Ludmila, Olga Herbenová, and Milena Lamarová (translated by Claudia Rosoux). *Pictorial Encyclopedia of Fashion, The.* Crown Publishers, New York, 1968.

LaBarre, Kathleen and Kay. *Reference Book of Children's Vintage Clothing: 1900–1919.* LaBarre Books, Portland, Oregon, 1996.

Larcom, Lucy. *A New England Girlhood.* Houghton, Mifflin, and Co., Boston, 1889.

Laubner, Ellie. *Fashions of the Roaring 20s.* Schiffer Publishing, Atglen, Pennsylvania, 1996.

Laver, James. *Children's Fashions of the 19th Century.* B.T. Batsford, London, 1951.

Lencek, Lena, and Gideon Bosker. *Making Waves.* Chronicle